"Clearly and sensitively written, this outstanding book is an important contribution to achieving long-term weight loss for the gastric bypass surgery patient. Ms. Peck has deep compassion, respect and understanding of the lives of the morbidly obese."

Dr. Alexander Sinclair
Beverly Hills, CA

"This is an extraordinary book with wisdom and insight on every page. Paula F. Peck has produced a remarkably practical and very readable volume. It is a veritable roadmap, or better, a complete travel guide for those on the journey toward health and wholeness via bariatric surgery. Written with charm, humor and compassion Exodus from Obesity is must reading for everyone considering weight loss surgery."

Dr. William G. Bixler
Clinical Psychologist
Manassas, VA

Exodus From Obesity

The Practical Guide to Successful Weight Loss After Surgery

Paula F. Peck, R.N.

BP Publishing books may be purchased for educational, business, or sales promotional use. For information, please write to: peckpublishing@yahoo.com

Library of Congress Control Number: 2003114984

Peck, Paula

Exodus, From, Obesity: The Guide to Long-Term Success After Weight Loss Surgery/Peck, Paula

ISBN 0-9728050-0-1

Cover photo by Jennifer Peck-Gonzalez.
Cover design by Trish McEachern.

Dedication

Two people share this dedication.

The first is to my sister, Dorothy Marian Slansky, who suffered from the disease of morbid obesity from her infancy and ultimately died from it. You were my mentor, so wise, intelligent and loving. You taught me music, to play guitar and to harmonize songs, which we sang together with all our hearts. You taught me to look at life as a running commentary of the foibles of the human race and we laughed until we ached. And from you I learned to be generous of spirit. You live forever in my memories as the consummate teacher, the older sister that I idolized and as my friend. This book is for you, Dottie.

The second dedication is to my daughter, Jennifer Peck-Gonzalez. In helping me edit this book, Jennifer, you relived the painful experience of having a morbidly obese mother. It wasn't easy to live with a mother who was constantly struggling for her health. Thank you for your straight arrow honesty all these years, for wisdom that astounds me over and again, for the courageous way you go about life and for the rock solid reliability of your support and friendship. You have been my deep pride and joy since I was twenty and having you for a daughter has made me happy. Indeed, it makes my heart dance just to know that I can call you mine. This book is for you, Jennifer.

Paula Felice Peck, November 2003

Author's Note

Eighty percent of the people who undergo gastric bypass surgery are women. For that reason and for the sake of readability, unless otherwise stated, when the feminine gender is used, both men and women are included where it is appropriate. Likewise, whenever the masculine gender is used, both men and women are included.

Contents

Opening 1

Chapt 1   My Road 3

Chapt 2   Deciding On Weight Loss Surgery 11

Chapt 3   Decision Made: The Initial Process For Surgery 23

Chapt 4   Preparing Emotionally For Weight Loss Surgery 31

Chapt 5   The Physical Process of Weight Loss Surgery 41

Chapt 6   After Surgery: Your Honeymoon Period 53

Chapt 7   3-6 Months After Surgery: Your Golden Period 65

Chapt 8   Six Months and Beyond: When Hunger Returns 79

Chapt 9   Overcoming Self-Defeat and Subterfuge 91

Chapt 10 Moving Through Space 103

Chapt 11 Navigating Through Food Landmines 123

Chapt 12 Dispelling Old Beliefs 141

Chapt 13 Dealing With Fat Prejudice 159

Chapt 14 Restructuring Relationships 165

Chapt 15 Adapting to Your New Image 173

Chapt 16 200 Pleasurable Things To Do Instead Of Eating. 183

Chapt 17 Celebrating Your New Life 191

Chapt 18 Sexual Feelings After Weight Loss 201

Chapt 19 Gratitude: Giving Something Back 209

Chapt 20 Containing Joy 215

Appendix 223

Bibliography 234

Exodus From Obesity

Opening

Let's imagine we are old friends seated in your living room, feet up, chatting and laughing. I am speaking to you, friend to friend, and sharing with you the information I have learned about obesity. I personally have experienced a weight loss of more than 175 pounds.... *twice* in my life.

To say that I know your life's pain from obesity would be disrespectful. I cannot know your particular life individually, but I do know about the isolation obesity imposes and the enormous emotional and physical pain it creates. I have fought this disease my entire adult life! As with most obese people, I had all the graduated sizes of clothes in my closet. I established my eating routines and rituals, and my obsessive feelings toward food lurked constantly right under the veneer of my skin.

Being a Registered Nurse and a Nationally Certified Massage Therapist, I had read volumes of information about health and disease including both Western and Eastern medicine and philosophies, but, in the end, unable to help myself, I sat down and wept for my life.

With all my other choices exhausted, I decided to have weight loss surgery. I lost 185 pounds. It is now almost five years later and I have maintained that weight loss and have a happy and healthy life. I am excited to share my experience with you.

If I can help you to succeed in your efforts with just one shred of information, if I can spare you some pain, if I can shine a light on a path that will assist your purpose in life to unfold, then I will be a friend.

Let's fly together...

Exodus From Obesity

[1]

My Road

"When you come to the edge of all the light you know and are about to step into the darkness of the unknown, faith is knowing that one of two things will happen: there will be solid ground to stand on, or you will be taught to fly."

– Author Unknown

Dottie and Me

There has never been a time in my life that I can remember where food and weight were not an issue.

My sister, Dottie, was obese as an infant, a child, an adolescent and an adult. She had become the major focus of our family and of my mother's endlessly nagging attempts to see her daughter thin.

My sister's life was centered around one diet attempt after another, all with varying degrees of initial success and, then, always failure. One such regimen that comes most painfully to mind was prescribed by a Beverly Hills physician who put Dottie on a diet consisting solely of diluted cream of corn soup. She followed this program for many months. Her weight plummeted to a dazzling 139 pounds. However, the minute she began eating normally, her weight soared to well over 200 pounds again. She had no time to enjoy her success.

Finally, in 1975, Dottie, at age 36, chose to undergo the Jejuno-Ileal Bypass Surgery. This type of surgery had so many complications it is rarely performed today. Those were the wild and wooly days of weight loss surgeries, it seems.

Her weight dipped again to 140 pounds and she assumed she was "home free." However, after 14 months, she began vomiting all day long. Her surgeon suggested, "Let's ride it out", and so she went home. She continued vomiting everything she ingested. The end result was an ambulance ride to the hospital with my sister in a coma. Her intestines were riddled with holes and her kidneys were scarred. Her laboratory findings were incompatible with human life. Dottie's internist slept at her bedside for two days to care for her. He was afraid that if he went home, Dottie would die.

To recover, she underwent a reversal of the original surgery, but her kidneys were destroyed forever.

The next three years brought Dottie dialysis and eight different surgeries, the last one of them an early stomach stapling procedure. She felt it would help her lose the regained weight that now made dialysis so painful. Before this last surgery she turned to me and said, "I've been thin and I've been fat. I'd rather be dead than fat again."

A prophesy of the coming event. Soon thereafter, her general condition was so compromised that her stomach ruptured and she died from blood poisoning at age 39.

My Journey

My journey was a struggle to overcome the pain and prejudice of obesity. At the age of 42, I weighed 311 pounds. I tore my entire life down in desperation. I left a nursing management position in a hospital department I helped to create. I put my California house on the market for sale, and my 14-year-old son and I moved to Durham, North Carolina.

Durham, known to those who resided there as "Fat City," was a comfortable Mecca for the obese. At that time in Durham, there were five major weight loss program centers. They offered fresh hope that an extreme attempt at weight loss would be the last one needed.

I rented an apartment, enrolled my son in school and entered a program for weight loss and lifestyle change. The program was at a school teaching addiction theory, exercise, nutrition, behavioral change, time management and stress management, among other topics. It offered group and individual therapy. It was their aim to attack weight problems from every angle they knew of, and the education proved invaluable to me.

I became my usual perfectionist taskmaster. I plopped myself down with the owner of the program, a psychologist, and I asked, "What is the profile of the people who are successful?"

Provided the factors for success, they became my roadmap, which I followed to the letter for the next 18 months. At the end of that journey I had lost 176 pounds and I wore a size 6. I even agreed to give a videotaped interview for the school to use in promoting its weight loss program. It satisfied my desire to offer hope to the newly entering people.

The remainder of that year and into the next, I underwent eight plastic surgeries, recovering sufficiently from one to face the next.

I struggled, "white-knuckling" weight maintenance for four years. I felt my body was screaming for food. Then, in the summer of 1996, many emotional events converged and I sought food as my solace again. In September, my mother died and my rapid return to obesity began in earnest. Finally, in 1999, I was desperate. I weighed 325 pounds and my health was deteriorating.

Searching for a way to end my misery, I followed the progress of a friend of mine who had undergone the Roux-en-Y Gastric Bypass weight loss surgery procedure nine months earlier. At times, as I observed his success, I was hoping to be granted the surgery myself. At other times, I was hoping to be dissuaded from the decision. In the midnight of my soul, I wondered if death would grant me a respite from the excruciating pain of obesity.

Every Monday would bring the "good girl" promise to diet. I would start a regimen in the morning and abandon it by noon. I knew in my heart that I simply did not have one more diet scheme left in me. My mood was angry, resentful and desperate.

I begged my friends to talk me out of weight loss surgery, pleading, "If you can think of any other way I can lose weight again and regain my health, please tell me."

They had no answers for me.

Finally, in March 1999, I made the decision to have the Roux-en-Y Gastric Bypass Surgery. I flew from Cape Cod, then my home, to California with a friend. Of course, I thought of Dottie constantly on the trip. Would I cause further injury to my health? Would I succumb to her fate and die a painful death? Would my children lose their mother? Facing the terror of possible death, it took all of my faith to face the task at hand.

I gained solace from reading and repeating a quote I had brought with me:

"When you come to the edge of all the light you know and are about to step into the darkness of the unknown, faith is knowing that one of two things will happen: there will be solid ground to stand on, or you will be taught to fly."

Somehow that faith sustained me.

My surgery went well. I awoke from the operation with the realization that I had been granted another chance at life.

I am about to celebrate the fifth anniversary of my surgery. My body has shed 185 pounds. I have found a renewed love of life. I am endlessly grateful.

I will embrace anyone who wants to walk through the door marked *Weight Loss Surgery*! I know of no other method that offers as much quality of life for the morbidly obese.

I will show you the road I took.

The journey is yours.

[2]

Deciding On Weight Loss Surgery

"And the day came when the risk to remain tight in the bud was more painful than the risk it took to blossom."

– Anais Nin

"Obesity is the most common form of malnutrition in the Western world."[1] "Every day, 25 percent of the United States population begins a diet. Even with the help of a diet industry worth about $30 billion a year, 95 percent of those who manage to shed unwanted pounds will regain them."[2]

"Your life is important. An eating disorder has thwarted it. The disorder has interrupted your thinking, distracted your purposes, stolen many of your hours and, quite possibly, it has also stolen chances, relationships and opportunities. I believe with all my heart that you have special, unique contributions only you can give to the world. I believe experiences are waiting for you that are especially for you. Your life has meaning. You may have lost track of what that meaning is, but it is there for you and you can find it again."[3]

Sowing the Seeds for Morbid Obesity

Obesity has been our pain and our sanctuary.

We suffer the emotional and physical wear and tear of daily life in an overweight body, this is true. And we wish our lives could be rid of that burden. We adapted originally as children, by choosing food as our coping mechanism. There we found solace from our emotional pain.

"Members of the bariatric and psychological communities have noted that a significantly high number of women (up to 85%) who are severely obese have been victims of abuse. The most frequent form is childhood sexual abuse. Neglect, poverty, parental mental illness, multiple stepparents or caretakers, parental alcoholism or drug use, as well as physical battering, rape and emotional abuse have also been reported. Individuals may eat in response to these abusive experiences to soothe themselves or stuff down frightening feelings."[4]

Weren't we smart little children to have found a way to survive the pain of childhood? Food became our protection, not the best of coping mechanisms, but what a child's mind could manage.

As adults, however, we no longer need to overeat as a method to cope with these painful feelings.

Inevitably, obese people get to the stage where the food no longer covers the considerable emotional pain. It has been said that the best day in the life of an addict is the first day of addiction with ever-decreasing reward after that. The cold day comes when the substance is unable to mask the pain any longer. Food, which seems a friend, now lets us down. So we must find healthier methods for dealing with our pain.

After surgery, make no mistake about it, there is often a grieving period for food. Part of that grieving is for the coping quality it gave to painful memories. The work of recovery is in dealing with these buried feelings and events without using food as the bandage to place over the wound. By dealing with the underlying pain, we heal.

"Obesity is a growing public health problem that affects 97 million American adults—55 % of the population."[5]

Obesity is a progressive illness. It is an increase in weight, year after year, mounting immobility and death 10 to 15 years earlier than people of normal weight.

"It is the second leading cause of preventable death in this country narrowly behind smoking, and it claims over 300,000 lives annually."[6]

"The risk of diabetes has been reported to be about twofold in the mildly obese, fivefold in moderately obese and *tenfold* in severely obese persons. The duration of obesity is also an important determinant of the risk for developing diabetes. The risk of developing diabetes also increases with age, if a family history is present and if the obesity is central.

Cancer mortality rates are increased in severely obese females; e.g., endometrium (5.4 times), gallbladder (3.6 times), uterine cervix (2.4 times), breast (1.5 times). Cancer mortality rates are increased in severely obese males; e.g., colorectum (1.7 times) and prostate (1.3 times)."[7]

In summary, we are a fat nation getting fatter, and diets don't solve the very real problem of a genetic disease coupled with a sedentary lifestyle.

We have been given the wrong tools with which to fight. The diets have failed us, not the other way around.

Morbid Obesity Is A Disease – Not A Failure of Willpower or Character

Morbid Obesity is a disease. Scientists have discovered there are many genes that give us the tendency to be obese. These genes determine our propensity to store body fat and, as critically important, *to delay our sense of satiety.* Since the stomach can stretch to accommodate *two quarts* of food, you can see how much caloric damage can be accomplished during a binge before the body finally signals that our appetite is fully satisfied.

"Medically, the word morbid means causing disease or injury. Morbid Obesity is a serious disease process in which the accumulation of fatty tissue on the body becomes excessive and interferes with or injures the other bodily organs causing serious and life-threatening health problems, which are called *co-morbidities.*"[8]

"How do we know it's genetic? Numerous studies have established that there is a very powerful genetic predisposition to Morbid Obesity:

- Children adopted at birth show no correlation of their body weight with that of their adoptive parents, who feed them and teach them how to eat. They show an 80% correlation of their body weight with their genetic parents, whom they have never even met.

- Identical twins, with the same genes, show a much higher similarity of body weights than do fraternal twins, who have different genes.

- Certain genetic populations, such as the American Indians of the Southwest, have a very high incidence of severe obesity. They also have a markedly increased incidence of diabetes and heart disease.

- There has never been a scientific study which has shown that dietary management is beneficial or effective in the severely obese."[8]

The Co-Morbidities of Obesity

The consequences of obesity are considerable. Here's a list of the co-morbidities of obesity:

- Accident Proneness
- Amenorrhea
- Angina Pectoris
- Ankle Pain
- Anxiety Disorder
- Back Pain
- Body Odor (severe)
- Breast Cancer
- Bronchitis
- Cervical Disk Disease
- Chest Pain
- Chronic Lower Extremity Swelling
- Chronic Neck Pain
- Cirrhosis
- Colon Cancer (males)
- Coronary Insufficiency
- Deep Venous Thrombosis
- Depression
- Diabetes Mellitus
- Difficult Intubation for Surgery
- Difficulty Walking
- Dysmenorrhea
- Economic Problems
- Enlarged Liver
- Excess Hair on Face (women)
- Excessively Heavy Menstruation
- Fatigue
- Foot Pain
- Gallstones
- Gastric Reflux Disease
- Gastritis
- Glucose Intolerance
- Gout
- Heart Muscle Disease
- Heel Spurs
- Hernias

- Hip Pain
- Hypertension
- Increased Blood Lipids
- Increased Operative Risk
- Infertility
- Inflammation and infection under hanging abdominal skin
- Kidney Disease
- Knee Pain
- Leg Ulcers
- Lumbar Disk Disease
- Muscle Weakness
- Osteoarthritis
- Ovarian Cancer
- Physical Problems
- Prostate Cancer
- Pulmonary Embolus (blood clot to lungs)
- Shortness of Breath
- Skin Abscesses, Boils
- Skin Inflammations
- Sleep Apnea
- Social Problems
- Sudden Death
- Unable to Sleep Lying Down
- Urinary Stress Incontinence (women)
- Uterine Cancer
- Varicose Veins
- Weakness
- Wheezing

The body, trying with all its compensatory might to accommodate the progressive weight gain, breaks down and succumbs.

Obesity or Surgery

We have to make lifestyle changes, no matter what avenue we choose to lose weight. However, the statistics from different sources place the rate of weight regain with diet regimens alone at somewhere between 95 and 98%.

Haven't you experienced this regain from dieting efforts yourself?

If your decision is to try another diet, then this is the choice as I see it: obesity or surgery. To me, there doesn't seem much else to say about the efficacy of diets alone once we reach the point of *morbid obesity* – 100 pounds or more overweight.

"Unfortunately, exercise alone has not been shown to be an effective treatment for morbidly obese patients. In a very careful study of morbidly obese patients by Bhorntorp and colleagues, exercise alone did not produce either weight loss or a decrease in fat content.

Nor have drugs or other treatments proven effective for the morbidly obese. Various drug treatments have been tried in obese patients, but none has been demonstrated effective in producing significant weight loss *that is maintained.*

In conclusion, currently available non-surgical treatments for morbid obesity are neither safe nor effective.

The physiologic hazards of weight loss, followed by weight regain, are significant and may predispose to further weight regain. These psychological hazards include the loss of self-esteem due to repeated failure and a significant tendency for developing a *diet depression* during calorie restriction. All these methods have potential value as *part* of a comprehensive program for surgical patients."[9]

Weight Loss Surgery

On the other side of conventional weight loss methods are the major risks of gastric bypass surgery. *Gastric bypass weight loss surgery is major surgery.*

The risk of death is generally held to be 0.5%, about the same as for other surgeries. Obviously, the skill of the surgeon and the general health of the patient have a bearing on these results. The Appendix includes a list from the International Bariatric Surgery Registry, which is a compilation of statistics for complications within 30 days of surgical treatment for obesity.

Laparoscopic Gastric Bypass Surgery is a complex procedure requiring experience. Logically, it is perfected by a surgeon having performed hundreds of these cases. Sometimes prospective patients do not go far enough in questioning their doctors. Although they may inquire whether he performs the surgery laparoscopically, few patients ask about the number of cases the surgeon has performed. If the doctor has done only 5 such cases last year, it may be wise to seek the services of a surgeon who has performed a larger number of these surgeries. There is less risk of complications from the surgery when an obese patient is on the operating table for as little time as possible, which comes with the experience of the surgeon. Inquire how the surgeon was trained and how many such cases he has done. You are wise and within your rights to ask the doctor his surgical statistics, e.g., death rate, infection rate, rate of leaks, etc. Ask who takes call for him after business hours? Will you know the doctor he refers you to?

Required Lifestyle Changes After Surgery

The Roux-en-Y Gastric Bypass surgery is a potent *tool* to make your lifestyle changes much easier. But remember, you will be getting a gastric bypass, not a *personality* bypass. You must commit to making changes in your behavior, your attitude and in your conceptual thinking. If you decide upon surgery with the intention of reversing it after you lose the weight, or if you are unwilling to commit to the lifestyle changes necessary to provide your body the best nutrition and health to maintain the weight loss, my best advice is *don't have the surgery.*

The investment you must make in your future is to commit to eating for proper nutrition. Since only a limited amount of food can fit in your pouch, and since the surgery creates some minor malabsorption of nutrients, you need to make sure that what you eat is of good nutritional quality.

You will *not* be dieting, but merely committing to a manner of eating that favors good nutrition and satiety. Now eating means starting your meal with a protein food first, then a vegetable, then fruit. Your carbohydrates will be obtained mostly from vegetables and fruit, much of which burn slower than refined carbohydrates and definitely offer greater nutrition. Add exercise to your life and you will have a health program whereby you can be of normal weight and healthier for life.

You No Longer Have to Accept the Minimum

There is a Sufi saying that goes –

> "*You have been invited to the Divine Banquet of Life and here you are crawling after crumbs.*"

Indeed, I feel we have been created to celebrate our lives and to move in a body free of encumbrances, so why are we settling for so little and "crawling after crumbs?" If we want our spirit to soar, our body must go with it. They are not separate.

We did not go to bed one night weighing 120 pounds and wake up at 350 pounds. The weight crept on as day by day we tolerated more and more physical and emotional pain. Eventually, we learned to accept what Anne Katherine in *Anatomy of an Addiction* described as the "Minimum".

"Most of us are probably well acquainted with having the minimum of something important. Minimum parenting, minimum attention, minimum boundaries, minimum assistance as children, minimum sanity in the environment, minimum safety, minimum reason to trust, minimum love or respect.

If you received minimal emotional support growing up, you are very familiar with deprivation.

Deprivation of emotional needs is abusive and harmful. It creates long-standing difficulties in later life and has consequences that reach far into the future."[3]

Now the challenge is to trust that you no longer must be crawling after the crumbs of life, that you can create both a soaring spirit and a body that will go along. Just as the trapeze artist must let go of one trapeze to grasp the next, we must have faith that in letting go of the old life we can create a new one. You deserve the color and abundance that life offers. Don't settle for less.

ACTION LIST:

➢ Attend support group meetings. Meet other people who are farther along in the process. Learn as much as you can.

➢ Attend seminars that give you information about the surgery and allow you to get an initial impression about the surgeon.

---

[3]

Decision Made:
The Initial Process For Surgery

"I took the road less traveled by, and that has made all the difference."

– Robert Frost   (Road Not Taken)

Once you have decided to go forward with surgery, commitment and patience are needed to reach your surgery date. It isn't easy to fight for yourself when you are at top weight and feeling poorly physically and in spirit. Muster all the strength you have and be committed to obtaining health insurance approval for gastric bypass surgery. For some patients, the process is smooth, short and easy, but for others it takes fortitude.

Generally, the process goes like this:

Calculate your Body Mass Index (BMI)—The BMI is a measure of the extent a person is overweight. It is calculated by dividing one's weight in kilograms by their height in meters squared. The Appendix includes a chart that makes that determination easy.

A BMI of 40 or above is the criterion given by the National Institutes of Health as candidacy for weight loss surgery. A BMI of 35 or above, with accompanying co-morbidities such as diabetes, hypertension, etc., are usually considered as justification for surgery by many insurance companies.

The National Institutes of Health established the following guidelines for considering patients for weight loss surgery. Patients should:

- "Be at least 100 pounds overweight.

- Have a co-morbidity that will be improved by the surgery.

- Be intelligent enough to understand the surgery and risks.

- Have no glandular problems causing their obesity.

- Have tried to lose weight by conventional means.

- Be willing to be observed over a long period of time."[10]

From the chart, find your BMI. Is yours in the range that is considered morbidly obese? If so, call your insurance company to see if it will cover gastric bypass surgery for morbid obesity. Each policy differs within a given insurance company. You need to determine what your specific policy allows. The term *morbid obesity* is crucial to the insurance company's decision. You have to speak their language.

If your insurance covers the surgery, call and schedule an appointment with your surgeon. If not, consider paying out of pocket yourself. Many medical practices offer finance plans. Maybe you could pay off a loan for surgery with the money you save on food each month? Did you ever calculate how much you spend on food every month? Or, maybe you could start a savings plan for plastic surgery later.

I know of an attorney whose law practice deals with obtaining insurance coverage for gastric bypass surgery patients. Often he can handle your problem over the phone or by e-mail. Contact me by e-mail (paula@paulapeck.com) if you need his name.

Even if you are denied insurance coverage, please don't assume that an appeal won't work. It does take tenacity, but by one way or another, find the way to prevail.

I advise speaking with prior patients for their experiences in dealing with doctors, reading Internet sites of the various medical practices considered, and going to the introductory seminars of the physicians best suited to you. Ask questions. Get as much education as possible. I find patients now are quite sophisticated in their knowledge of the procedure. They have been "shopping".

Call your surgeon's office and make an appointment for an initial consultation. Ask the nurse to send an information packet and a health questionnaire to your home. Fill out the questionnaire thoroughly and bring it with you to your first visit or mail it back to the surgeon's office after retaining a copy for yourself. It is worth the time taken with this lengthy list of questions. From your answers, the nurse or insurance verifier in your doctor's office creates a letter to your insurance company for insurance approval.

Meet with your doctor and get an impression of him and of the staff in his office. Unlike other types of surgeries the doctor might perform, gastric bypass surgery puts him in continuing relationship with you for at least a year afterward, and he must be dedicated to your long-term follow up care. If you can't confide in him without receiving negative judgment, I would not consider him a good choice. Look for a compassionate soul, as well as a talented surgeon.

Ask about the "program" he offers. You will need an educational program providing you classes before surgery and after. Hopefully, his practice offers a support group where you can share your feelings, fears and triumphs, and, where you can obtain information on the many new skills you must build.

Did you know you are allowed to request a particular anesthesiologist when your surgery is booked? Ask your surgeon who he thinks works best with gastric bypass patients. Ask the office nurse to call the surgery department of the hospital to request your choice of anesthesiologist.

The preparatory requirements for surgery vary, but generally you will have laboratory work done on a sample of your blood, a chest x-ray, an upper GI study and an EKG. Some surgeons ask for cardiac studies, abdominal ultrasound and sometimes a pelvic ultrasound done pre-operatively. Due to the insurance company's demand, they also require a psychological exam to identify individuals who would not be good surgical candidates due to the fact they would not comply with the regimen afterwards. Your doctor also wants to know you understand what life will be like post-operatively without illusions.

The factor that usually prolongs this process is in the waiting for approval from your insurance company. Be patient. The wait is worth it.

In the Psychological Aspects of Gastric Bypass Surgery, Erica Wald writes:

"Even though a significant weight loss lessens numerous medical problems, many patients list social rather than medical considerations as their reason for requesting surgery. The psychological outcomes of gastric bypass surgery include: decrease in social prejudice and discrimination, improvement in eating behavior, decrease in body image disparagement, increase in self-esteem, increased activity and improvement in social relationships."[11]

Reviewing this quote may help sustain you through the waiting period.

Also noteworthy, "Over 95% of all weight-related health problems (co-morbidities) such as high blood pressure, diabetes, sleep apnea, gastroesophageal reflux, stress incontinence, and degenerative arthritis pain, are relieved by one year after the operation - often much sooner."[8]

With all the study results back to your surgeon and the approval from your insurance company in hand, his office schedules your surgery with the hospital.

Pregnancy Issues

If you decide on the Roux-en-Y Gastric Bypass Surgery now, you should be informed that while you will be able to nourish a healthy pregnancy later on, it is not advisable to become pregnant for at least 12 months post-operatively and many doctors feel you should wait up to two years. Many morbidly obese women begin ovulating again after they have the surgery. Birth control measures are necessary to prevent a pregnancy. Give yourself a chance to adjust to the many changes that gastric bypass surgery imposes upon your body. Those first two years are a time for you to lose a tremendous amount of weight, to have your body heal and adjust and to work on the emotional factors of your life. It is your time.

ACTION LIST:

➤ Find your BMI on the chart provided.

➤ Call your insurance company to see if your policy covers gastric bypass surgery for morbid obesity.

➤ Think about a plan for alternate coverage if your insurance does not allow for this surgery.

➤ Call your surgeon's office for an appointment.

➤ Read the information packet from your surgeon and complete the health questionnaire.

➤ On your first visit to your surgeon have a written list of your questions and concerns. Also include a list of your allergies and of the medications and dosages you are currently taking.

➤ Bring a loved one with you to the first consultation. When you are nervous it is hard to remember everything that is explained to you.

➤ After your consultation, go to a quiet place with peaceful surroundings to be alone and to think. After all, this surgery is a life-altering event. No on can force you to have surgery. Come to your final decision about gastric bypass surgery with your mind resolute and with peace in your heart.

[4]

Preparing Emotionally For Weight Loss Surgery

"The wind, one brilliant day, called."

– Antonio Machado

"The flower sheds all its petals and finds the fruit."

– Tagore (Fireflies)

Who Am I Now? My "Dear Me Letter"

As I began my journey from obesity, I found it helpful to evaluate what my life had become. I asked myself, "Who am I now?"

I answered that question by creating a *"Dear Me Letter."*[12] This was a letter only to myself. Its purpose was to be an inspirational guide both through the surgery and afterward. In this letter, before my surgery, I described what my life was like and how frightened I was to begin an exercise program at 325 pounds so I could prepare for the surgery. How far would I be able to walk before I couldn't return? What if someone had to come to help me? How would they get me home? These worries and many others plagued me, such as aching joints, shin splints and thighs that rubbed raw.

I wrote how my son, as I drove him to his junior high school, begged me to drop him off a block away from the school. It wasn't hard to guess he was embarrassed to have a morbidly obese mother.

My daughter would tell me in later years, "Mom, at that time, I just figured you would die early, so I thought I would love you all I could before you left me."

My children were more savvy and aware of my condition than credit was given.

I wrote, further, how unprepared I was for the opportunities that came my way, and I judged them on the basis of whether I could manage them physically or whether I thought I might be embarrassed if I tried to do them.

I knew that merited job promotions did not come easily. I had to fight for them, and I'm sure that I was overlooked at times because of my "image."

I revealed that I drove up to a pharmacy one day when I needed cough drops for a cold. I then realized that the item I wanted was in the rear of the store. I sat in the car quite a while, determining whether it would be worth the pain of walking all the way to the back of the store to make my purchase. Tears came to my eyes when I realized how contracted and burdened my life had become.

I have had more than one door slammed in my face by a man who didn't feel that holding it open for a "fat" woman was worth his time. And I felt hurt and slighted when I saw bumper stickers that read, "No Fat Chicks."

In short, I confided in my letter that I felt either held up to ridicule or rendered invisible in a world that looked right past me. "If only people could see the real me inside," I would cry.

That, and more, was the content of my *Dear Me Letter*.

Now I ask you to have the courage to look your life squarely in its face and to write your own description of how it is to live in your body today. The tears that it may bring will mark the beginning of a process of recognition and the road to recovery.

Remember, this is a letter only to *yourself* to inspire you both through the surgery, if you choose it, and afterward. About six months after surgery, when your hunger returns, modifying your eating habits will be frustrating. We miss our food rituals and romanticize about the "old days".

When you review your *Dear Me Letter*, you will remember why you embarked on this journey in the first place, and patience and gratitude will sweep over you.

You will find caring people on your path to offer instruction, inspiration and hope. I will help you all I can.

Education and Support

Preparing emotionally for weight loss surgery allays your fears, reduces pain, minimizes depression and builds self-confidence.

Look for a surgeon who has created educational and support programs for his patients. You will have many questions both before and after your surgery. The program should consist of:

- Knowledgeable and compassionate nurses on his staff to answer your questions.

- Follow-up care for one year by your surgeon.

- Educational classes that include both pre-operative and post-operative information.

- A support group that meets *regularly* to provide you a forum in which to share experiences, to get your questions answered, to become educated and to provide a social outlet. As obesity progresses, we tend to isolate ourselves. A support group offers social stimulation and a way to turn away from food and towards relationships with people, instead.

With the myriad emotional changes that will occur from rapid weight loss, an appointment with a psychologist knowledgeable in weight issues can smooth your transition, as well.

The Surgical Athlete

Here is a challenge for you that I give prospective surgical candidates: *Become a surgical athlete!* By this I mean go into an active training mode for your upcoming event. You may think of yourself as too tired or sick to do anything, but there are numerous actions you can take to prepare yourself mentally and physically for your operation.

➢ With your doctor's approval, begin a walking program now to improve respiratory and cardiovascular health and to introduce the habit of walking which you'll continue after surgery. Begin by walking first to the mailbox, then halfway down the street, progressing farther each day, or practice walking in a shallow pool for minimal impact upon joints.

➢ Many times a day, take a series of 10 full deep breaths, filling your lungs, holding the breath and then exhaling. Deep breathing increases the capacity of the lungs.

➢ Start taking a multi-vitamin and a calcium supplement daily.

➢ At meals, eat protein first, then vegetable, then fruit.

➢ Drink plenty of water.

➢ Do not take aspirin or aspirin products, gingko biloba, garlic tablets, ginger tablets, or Feverfew within two weeks of your surgery. They delay the time it takes for your blood to clot. Avoid Ephedra, Kava-Kava and St. John's Wort, as well, as they affect the cardiovascular system.

➢ Have someone take a "before" picture of you.

➢ Write your *Dear Me Letter* and tuck it away.

➢ Create the most positive mental framework you can. Imagine your life improving steadily day by day until your dreams are met. Close your eyes and imagine yourself in the room in which you would like to be seated. What does it look like? Imagine your body rising above the room, and picture the home you would like to be living in. Now ascend further and imagine the community in which you would like to reside. Who are the people with you there? What are you doing for work there? Can you envision yourself a person of normal weight, healthy, happy, laughing and surrounded by loving people? Ascend further and view the part of the world your community is in. Surround yourself with musical sound that touches your heart, with the beauty of nature and envision a full spectrum of color.

➢ This is a good time for a spiritual connection that is personal and meaningful to you. Your spiritual counselor can lend guidance and support in this anxious time.

As you can see, you are not merely a passenger along for the ride of surgery, but an active driver of your own fate, a surgical athlete.

A Final Pigout

I am *not* advocating stringent dieting when I suggest you become a surgical athlete. I am merely giving you an option to establish the healthy habits you will need to develop after surgery for maintaining your weight loss long-term. Since a new habit needs about three weeks to become a part of us, why not start now? It will raise your self-esteem, as well, to be doing something each day for your body, your mind and your spirit.

I think it appropriate to add a word about the last "pigout." Having made the suggestion to become a surgical athlete to a prospective patient one day, she seemed to like the idea. She said she would become one before surgery to decrease possible complications.

Another nurse, however, spoke with this patient later and told her, "I regret that I didn't have a pigout before my own surgery." The patient went home and proceeded to go on a regimen of ice cream for an entire week prior to her operation.

When a patient has an enlarged, fat-infiltrated liver, it makes laparoscopic surgery more difficult. The surgeon must get up under the liver to reach the stomach.

Some surgeons, upon seeing a greatly enlarged liver on an ultrasound, will place their patients on a diet of clear liquids for a few days before surgery. This reduces some of the fatty deposit in the liver.

So, can you imagine what got deposited into the liver of this woman who ate nothing but high fat ice cream for a solid week before surgery? She certainly wasn't making the situation easier on her surgeon or on herself. She wasn't establishing good nutrition so she could heal afterwards, plus she was psychologically preparing herself for a feeling of deprivation and program failure later.

So, envision yourself a surgical athlete and train for "gold."

ACTION LIST:

➢ Write your own *Dear Me Letter.*

- Reflect on how your life is impacted by your current body size.

- Describe how it is to live in your body.

- How do you fit into theatre seats?

- What is it like to fit in an airplane seat?

- What do your children tell their friends about you?

- Do you contemplate whether a chair will hold your weight before you sit down?

- Do your joints ache?

- Are you short of breath?

- Describe your mood, self-esteem, body image, social life, health problems, appearance and mobility.

- Include the prejudice you feel by being obese in our obsessively thin society.

The Physical Process of Weight Loss Surgery

"You have to leave the city of your comfort and go into the wilderness of your intuition....What you'll discover will be wonderful. What you'll discover will be yourself."

Alan Alda, "Dig into Life," Reader's Digest, May 1981

The Physical Experience

When I was investigating weight loss surgery for myself, I read about the many options available. It seemed inconceivable to me to consider having parts of my digestive system cut and rerouted elsewhere. After all, God hadn't hooked me up that way. I made my decision based on getting the best help for my disease with the least malabsorption of nutrients. My goal was not just a change in appearance, but a quest for robust health, as well.

The *Roux-en-Y Gastric Bypass* is considered the "gold standard" against which other surgical options are measured, and 80% of people having weight loss surgery have the Roux-en-Y Gastric Bypass.

For that reason, I have chosen not to discuss other surgical options. I learned all surgeries offer tradeoffs. I chose the Roux-en-Y because it allows for restriction of food ingested, provides early appetite satiety, has the least malabsorption of nutrients and, in addition, causes dumping, which limits sugar intake.

As in all new endeavors in life at that time, I focused much of my worry and concern about possible circumstances and outcomes that never transpired. The expression "the anticipation is worse than the realization" was certainly apt. Little negative was realized, my slight complications were easily handled, discomfort was dealt with and forgotten, and I had a good outcome.

The knowledge of possible problems is paramount to good decision-making, but the constant dwelling on possible problems causes unnecessary anxiety and debilitates health. Hopefully, the following will give you the basic knowledge you need to alleviate some of your anxiety.

What Is Gastric Bypass Surgery?

Briefly, here is what is accomplished with the gastric bypass: "In Gastric Bypass Surgery, the stomach is completely stapled shut and the outlet of the pouch opens into the intestine rather than into the rest of the stomach. This is done by dividing the small bowel just beyond the duodenum and bringing it up to the pouch to construct a connection. The other open end of the bowel is sewn back into the side of the Roux limb of intestine, completing the Y-shaped arrangement that gives the technique its name.[13]" [Named after Dr. Cesar Roux.]

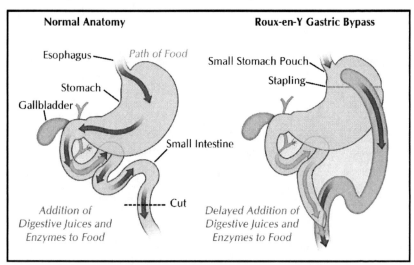

Figure 1 Digestive System
(The Journal of the American Medical Association)

The results from this procedure are:

- You will be able to eat only about an ounce of food (about the size of your thumb) at each meal in the early months.

- You will feel full quickly.

- The Dumping Syndrome will limit your intake of sweets.

To perform Gastric Bypass Surgery, a general surgeon takes advanced training in bariatric surgery. ("Baros" is the Greek word for weight.)

There are two methods for entering the body for the Roux-En-Y Gastric Bypass Surgery. The earlier method known as a *laparotomy* makes a surgical opening down the abdomen.

The later method, performing Roux-En-Y *laparoscopically,* involves making approximately six openings of one-half inch each into the abdomen and inserting instruments attached to a video monitor or headset for viewing. A skillful, experienced surgeon can complete the surgery in around one to two hours, often closer to the one-hour mark.

Internally, the surgery is the same for either approach.

However, with the laparoscopic approach there is generally less discomfort, less scarring and a shorter stay in the hospital. Also most laparoscopy patients can return to work earlier than with the open laparotomy procedure.

The Day Before Surgery

This would be a good time to record your physical measurements, to weigh yourself and to have a "before" picture taken. This is the last time you will see yourself at this weight and with these measurements. All pictures, weights and measurements from here on will be so much better, so take heart.

The regimen for the day before surgery varies slightly from surgeon to surgeon, but basically, the following is true: all your questions about the procedure should now have been answered. You are aware of the life changes that the Gastric Bypass Surgery imposes and what is expected of you post-operatively. Laboratory tests, chest x-ray, EKG and other studies have been completed. You have purchased, in advance, the necessary post-operative foods you require, in accordance with your surgeon's instructions, so they are waiting for you upon your return home from the hospital. You have obtained prescriptions for pain medication and antibiotics ahead of time, if your doctor allows, and you have filled them before the surgery. If you have *sleep apnea*, you have discussed with your surgeon the feasibility of bringing your CPAP machine with you to the hospital.

Many surgeons will allow you to have your *last* pre-operative solid meal for breakfast today and, then, a clear liquid diet consisting of Jell-O®, broth and water. Most doctors require you to take laxatives to clear the bowel. Follow your doctor's instructions about taking any other medications.

Consume nothing by mouth, neither fluids nor food of any kind, after midnight. *This is very important.* Your digestive tract must be as cleared and as quiet as possible.

Congratulations on your courage. My very best wishes and prayers are with you. Please e-mail me and let me know your thoughts and experiences. My e-mail address is: paula@paulapeck.com.

Surgery Day – Pre-operative

For most cases, the regimen is to arrive at the hospital two hours before the time of surgery. Bring a written list of any medications and their dosages you are currently taking. You don't need to bring the actual medications, since your surgeon leaves an order for them to be filled by the nurse caring for you after surgery.

Also, bring a written list of any allergies you have to medications, tape, latex, or iodine, if you have had a prior negative reaction to anesthesia, or anything you can think of that has provoked an allergic reaction.

In the preparation room for surgery, the nurse starts an intravenous (IV) drip and gives you IV fluids and IV antibiotics. She asks you questions about your allergies and when you last ate or drank anything. These questions and others are asked by many individuals in the hospital as a crosscheck so that all necessary information is accurately entered on your chart and nothing needed for your care is overlooked. The nurse verifies your written consent for the surgery, making sure you understand what will be performed. If you have chosen the laparoscopic surgery as your procedure, you will sign a consent form permitting your surgeon to convert to an "open" laparotomy procedure, if it is necessary for your safe care.

If gallbladder disease is visualized on the ultrasound study, your surgeon may remove your gall bladder during the gastric bypass surgery. This is done because the subsequent weight loss afterwards can increase the formation of gallstones, necessitating further surgery later. All these possibilities are indicated on your written hospital consent.

When ready, you are transported on a rolling bed or gurney to a room outside of the operating room. Your anesthesiologist greets you there, and he will stay with you the entire time in the operating room to assist your breathing, to give you anesthesia and other medications, and to monitor your vital signs. He never leaves your side.

When I had surgery, I asked the anesthesiologist to play soothing music in the operating room and to talk to me from time to time, telling me I will have little pain, that I will heal well, and that I will awaken happy and energized. It has been suggested that patients who are soothed this way during surgery require less medication for pain afterwards.

At this point it is time to give hugs and kisses to your relatives. There is a special waiting room designated for them. You are wheeled into the operating room and assisted in sliding onto the surgery table. *You are about to begin a new life! Happy Birthday!*

Surgery Day – Post-operative

After your operation, you may be vaguely aware of your surroundings as you awaken in the Recovery Room. You may feel a bit wired up to signal another planet. The IV is hooked up to one arm, a blood pressure cuff is on the opposite arm. A small tube (catheter) is coming out of your bladder, (placed while you were asleep in surgery), and which is attached to a collection bag at the foot of your bed. A soft clothespin-type device placed on one of your fingers measures your blood oxygen level. Often there are pneumatic "leg squeezers" on your lower legs, which are soft cotton wraps that gently compress and release your legs intermittently so that blood is pumped back to your heart to prevent blood clots that could possibly travel to your lungs. And you may have an oxygen tube in your nose.

Here's a TIP about the urinary catheter: it can be uncomfortable. A major complaint is that it makes you feel as if you still have to urinate because it keeps the muscle around the neck of the bladder open all the time. The pressure of urine on the muscle is ordinarily your body's signal that your bladder has to be emptied. Relax and pretend you are going to let go and urinate in bed. It won't happen. The catheter will collect the urine, your bed will remain dry and you will be more comfortable.

Many hospitals use a Patient Controlled Analgesia (P.C.A.) device, which attaches to your IV and allows you to press a button to release a predetermined, controlled amount of pain medication into the IV tubing. It is calibrated to prevent you from overdosing on the pain medication. You are in control and you won't have to wait for a nurse to bring you an injection of pain medication. It is surprising how comfortable this system keeps you. Only you or the nurse, have the responsibility of pushing the button. It is not appropriate for any guest to push the button for you.

Much of how well you recover from the surgery depends on your willingness to assume responsibility for part of your care. Look to take an active role so you don't feel so dependent on others.

You may have an awareness of awakening in the Recovery Room or in your hospital room later on. Move around in bed, deep breathe and walk as soon as you can.

During the first 24 hours after surgery, you will feel uncomfortable, but the next day, you will be astounded at your improvement. Twenty-four hours in the life of a post surgical patient makes a significant difference. So allow yourself to look at healing as a process. Even if there are setbacks, *they* get better. Be patient. Each day brings improvement, and each day you are gaining more independence.

The Day Of Discharge — At Home

Usually, you can anticipate discharge from the hospital on the second day after surgery with the laparoscopic method or on the third or fourth day with the open incision method. This timeframe varies with the surgeon and, of course, with your health and self-sufficiency after surgery.

Finally you're home again. The transition from your hospital bed to your home is tiring and a nap is welcomed. Catnap and walk. They are your tasks. Walking is a great aid to recovery. Try to walk throughout the house, then outside, progressing to longer and longer sessions each day. Expect to tire very easily, often for weeks. Be patient with yourself.

After surgery, it is not unusual to feel depressed and to cry. The body has gone through a lot of changes and it needs to adapt. Initially, it is emotionally difficult for many people to conceive of having a very little stomach. "What have I done to myself?" is a familiar question. Sometimes we feel "Buyers Remorse." Later on, this feeling passes and there isn't the strange thought of having been "altered".

We perceive that we have lost our comfort, our solace and our "friend", food. There may be real grieving for food after surgery. This feeling is natural. As you will see, by feeding your body protein, taking your vitamins, walking in the fresh air and connecting spiritually, your life will be better than it ever was. Do something for your mind, your body and your spirit each day. Laugh often. And remember, you now have a support group to access for reassurance and understanding whenever you need it. Avail yourself of psychological counseling if you feel you need help through this period. Ask your priest, pastor, rabbi or other spiritual counselor to guide you and to provide comfort.

ACTION LIST:

In The Hospital After Surgery

➢ Take deep breaths every time you wake up, 10 at a time. This, admittedly, is not fun. Just do it. Every hour use the device given to you called the Incentive Spirometer. It helps to aerate your lungs.

➢ Ask the nurses to help you to get up the night of surgery and to stand by your bed. The sooner you start to move around the better.

➢ Pump your feet up and down in bed, to simulate walking. In the hospital, plan each day with two goals: rest and walking. Catnap often. Then walk around the ring of patient rooms at least 4-5 times a day.

At Home

➢ Take catnaps.

➢ Walk ever-increasing distances.

➢ Pay strict attention to nutritional intake.

➢ Sip water.

➢ Start a journal to chronicle your journey.

➢ Lighten your spirit by laughing a lot.

[6]

After Surgery:
Your Honeymoon Period

"Let a joy keep you. Reach out your hands and take it when it runs by."

– Carl Sandburg (1878 - 1967)

Immediately after surgery, your Honeymoon Period has begun.

You don't feel hungry and, during this period, you lose weight easily and quickly. Since you can only tolerate a small amount of food in your newly created pouch, which is irritable and not too distensible, you are eating less food less often.

It takes about three months for your pouch to heal completely. During the Honeymoon Period, think of your new stomach as you would a small baby. Protect it. Don't overload the pouch to test how much it will stretch. It is truly a miracle to be cherished.

If you look at your thumb and its knuckle, you get an idea of how little your stomach pouch is and how little it holds. As you learn new eating behaviors, it is imperative that your goal be to obtain good nutrition. Since you can't eat very much, make what you eat good quality food. Buy the very best food you can afford.

Your New Way of Eating

For several weeks after surgery, some surgeons allow you to ingest only protein shakes, while others allow you to eat food as soon as you are discharged from the hospital. Regardless, you are "feeling your way" as to how your new stomach will respond to what it is fed. The most important points to remember are: *eat a small bite and eat it slowly.* I can't stress enough the value of small portions, small plates, small bites and chewing your food well. It takes time to break the lifelong habit of eating fast. It takes mindfulness and continuous diligence.

In addition, it is uncomfortable to drink liquid *with* your food. Fluids make food swell. Instead of relieving an uncomfortable sensation, your discomfort increases when you drink liquids with your meal. You may feel like vomiting to gain relief. So, whatever you have eaten, if your pouch doesn't like it, water won't help.

One patient told me, "I am not the kitchen sink! Pouring water after food doesn't work."

Here are reasons not to drink for at least ½ hour before eating your meal:

- It makes the food swell and creates discomfort.

- It washes the food out of the stomach pouch earlier, which lessens the feeling of satiety.

- It fills up the pouch with water at a time when it is crucial to be putting nutritious food into it.

- It makes you feel full when you need to be sensing how much food needs to go into the pouch before you feel satisfied.

One-half to one hour after eating, it is important to start sipping water and to drink often, increasing the quantity. By "loading water," the filled Roux limb of your intestine signals the brain that you are no longer hungry.

A high water intake protects your kidneys from the tendency to form the crystals that cause kidney stones. Better weight loss is promoted by ridding your system of these waste products.

Vomiting

Continual vomiting may mean there is a stricture caused by scarring at the connection (anastomosis) of your intestine and pouch, usually occurring at the end of the first month. Report this situation to your doctor. Under mild anesthetic, as an outpatient procedure, this area can be dilated using an endoscope to relieve the stricture.

The Dumping Syndrome

The consumption of too much carbohydrate causes a condition that goes by the name of the *Dumping Syndrome*. What happens is that the swallowed food is passed along quickly to the intestines where it combines with insulin metabolizing it into glucose, a form of sugar. In that form it is able to be absorbed into the body. A potato, for example, contains a little over 50 grams of starch, which the digestive tract metabolizes into 50 grams of sugar, around a quarter of a cup.

Adding a quarter cup of sugar to the your existing blood level causes your blood sugar level to rise rapidly. In response, your pancreas dumps insulin, sometimes twice the normal amount, into the bloodstream, thus the origin of the name *Dumping Syndrome*.

When this happens, you feel sweaty and experience flu-like symptoms. You may feel sick to your stomach, have a rapid pulse, experience dizziness, show flushed skin, undergo a general sense of weakness and have a great desire to lie down and sleep. Not everyone experiences all of these symptoms. The reaction varies in intensity and lasts for about 20 to 60 minutes, although some people experience it longer. Then, it quickly goes away. This adverse reaction will cause you to think long and hard before ingesting sugary foods again.

Additionally, your liver converts sugar into fats when insulin levels are elevated.

After you "dump", your blood sugar will drop again and you will feel hungry! Suddenly hungry, you grab a quick food fix, usually another carbohydrate snack, and the sugar/insulin cycle begins again.

For many, the *Dumping Syndrome* occurs with the ingestion of more than 18 grams of sugar at a meal. Considering that *plain* yogurt has 16 grams of sugar per serving, it shows you how commonly manufacturers add sugar to our foods. Read labels carefully. They may surprise you.

These substances are forms of sugar:

- Beet Sugar
- Brown Sugar
- Cane Sugar
- Corn-Syrup Solids
- Dextrose
- Food Products Ending in *Ose* (except Cellulose)
- Fructose
- Glucose
- Honey
- Lactose
- Malto-Dextrin
- Mannitol® (alcohol that converts to sugar in the stomach)
- Maple Sugar or Syrup
- Molasses
- Rice Sugar

- Sorbitol® (alcohol that converts to sugar in the stomach)

- Sucrose

- Turbinado Sugar

These substances usually contain sugar:

- Alcoholic Beverages
- Bacon
- Bagel
- Barbeque Sauce
- Beef Broth (canned)
- Bologna
- Bouillon
- Bread
- Cereals
- Chicken Broth (canned)
- Cider
- Cold Cuts
- Cold Medicine (liquid)
- Corn (canned)
- Cough Drops
- Cough Syrup
- Crackers
- Cream Soups
- Cured Meat
- Dates
- Dinner Mixes
- Dried Fruit
- Equal®
- Fig
- Fish-Smoked
- Frozen Dinners
- Fruit Juice
- Fruits (canned)
- Frying Batter
- Gravies
- Juices (canned)
- Ketchup
- Marinade
- Meat-Smoked
- Milk-Flavored
- Pasta

- Peas (canned)
- Pizza Crusts
- Pizza Dough
- Processed Meats
- Round Beans (canned)
- Sandwich Buns

In most cases, the healthy nutrients from refined carbohydrates are stripped out of food and little is left, nutritionally. White bread, for instance, is advertised as having vitamins added to it. What the label doesn't tell is that many more vitamins are stripped out of the bread than are replaced, leaving the bread of diminished nutritional value.

These substances have *refined carbohydrates* that break down quickly into sugar:

- Dressing
- Frozen Yogurt
- Ham
- Hot Dog
- Potato Chips
- Salad
- Sauce Mix
- Sauces
- Sausage
- Some Fried Batters
- Spaghetti Sauce
- Sugar Twin®
- Sweet N' Low®
- Sweet-And-Sour Sauce
- Teriyaki
- Tofutti®
- White Bread

A Quick Sugar Reference

I use a table called a glycemic index. It tells me at a glance what foods have a high concentration of sugar. I have included some common foods that have medium-high (MH), high (H) and very high (VH) glycemic sources:

Apricots-MH	Flour-H
Bagel-H	Grits-H
Banana-H	Mango-MH
Biscuit-H	Millet-H
Bread sticks-H	Muffins-H
Bread-French-H	Oat bran-H
Bread-reduced calorie-H	Parsnips-H
Bread-rye-H	Pickles, sweet-H
Buns, hamburger-H	Pita-H
Carrots-H	Popcorn-VH
Cornbread-H	Potato, baked-VH
Corn-H	Potato, mashed-VH
Cornmeal-H	Raisins-H
Cranberry sauce-H	Rice cakes-VH
Croissant-H	Rice, brown-MH
Croutons-H	Spaghetti, wheat-MH
Dates-H	Waffles-H
Dinner roll-H	Wheat bread-H
Egg noodles-H	White bread-H
English muffin-H	Yam-MH

Carbohydrate Potholes

I often see patients falling into three potholes in the road concerning carbohydrates:

1. *Crunchy Foods.* I most commonly see patients revert to eating popcorn. We have been taught that popcorn is low in calories. You can see by the glycemic index, that popcorn has a very high factor. All of these high glycemic factor foods convert to sugar easily. Ostensibly, you are eating sugar when you snack on popcorn. It is much easier if you don't get in the habit of snacking on it in the first place, as it reinforces a connection between a negative event and the salving of feelings with food. Popcorn becomes soft in our mouths and slides down easily. It doesn't take long before large quantities are consumed.

TIP: When you look at dinner tonight, instead of saying, "I have chicken and vegetables and fruit on my plate," look at your food as, "I have a healthy portion of protein, a food high in Vitamin A and a small amount of food that has a medium glycemic factor." It isn't too appetizing, but isn't it interesting to look at food dispassionately and for what it will give you nutritionally? A different exercise in thinking, yes? Of course you won't see all your meals this way, and it is certainly OK to look forward to your food and to enjoy it, but we ordinarily eat in such an unconscious way that we really aren't looking at what the food will provide us.

2. *Unidentifiable Foods.* Casseroles fit this description. The problem is that we often don't know what's in them, nor the proportions of foods we do recognize. How much vital protein are you getting? Or, are you really loading up on carbohydrates? It is easier to stay on program if you can identify the food in its original form. A piece of barbequed chicken, for instance, looks

like a piece of raw chicken in form. You can judge portion size that way. Chicken in a pot pie looks like what?

3. *The Mighty Sandwich.* I have never met an obese person who didn't love sandwiches. I, myself, could skillfully load all the Thanksgiving foods between two slices of bread. You too? Sandwiches present more carbohydrates than the protein-to-carbohydrate ratio you need on your program. Especially in the early months after surgery when you need to get enough protein to heal, sandwiches leave a question as to how much good protein you are actually getting when you fill up on bread. Instead, you are consuming more carbohydrates and, therefore, more sugar.

Prevent Dumping – Eat Protein First

At each meal, eat protein foods *first,* then a vegetable, then some fruit. This program limits carbohydrates to the *third* item eaten, keeping your blood sugar in a more moderate zone and preventing dumping.

Take Pictures

Be sure to measure your success visually. In addition to Before Surgery pictures, take photos, monthly along the way and date them. It is exciting to see the differences in your image. Notice changes in your clothes. Record in your journal when you began to tuck in a shirt or when you could finally wear a belt, for instance. Remember, these are your milestones. Celebrate yourself! But not with food.

Record Measurements

Taking your measurements from time to time allows you to see your weight success in a different way. Muscle tissue is heavier than fat, so your progress isn't always reflected as a weight loss on the scale. You *are* losing fat though, and your clothes fit better and better.

ACTION LIST:

➤ Create a journal and chronicle your progress. Starting with pre-surgical days, chart your measurements to the end goal. Weight loss is uneven and plateaus occur. As motivation, measure the inches lost as well as pounds.

7

3-6 Months After Surgery: Your Golden Period

"Food is used for many purposes other than nutritional survival. It is used to soften up people socially, to sell houses, to manipulate business sales, to impress a date, to be a centerpiece for activities, to stabilize families and to unite a culture. In fact, food is probably used for psychological purposes more often than any other activity or substance.

For some of us, however, food is like a lifeline, an essential tool in our survival kit. It takes us away from stress, it numbs our fears and worries, and it stops the world and lets us get off. It's a womb, a haven, a cave, an escape and a refuge.

Eating is an automatic response to feelings—so quickly applied without thought—that breaking this pattern takes tremendous sustained effort. If food has become a cornerstone and the cornerstone is removed, an equally strong foundation must replace it.

With time, with an investment in your weight loss and with new habits of lifestyle, your mood lifts and life seems sweeter. The pain that eating had masked now is exposed and we no longer can use food to help us cope. The real work now, is in dealing with our pain without using food as an emotional bandage."

- Anatomy of a Food Addiction

Do you remember in elementary school the kid who could only eat one-quarter of a peanut butter sandwich and who then would toss the remainder aside? That person's body registered satiety early in the eating experience. Well, *you* have just joined the ranks of those people who feel satisfied with a small amount of food ingested early in a meal, as well. That's what you paid your money for, a *tool* that will allow you to eat less, comfortably, and to feel satisfied quickly with that amount.

Your Golden Period

Three to six months after surgery, the *Golden Period* as I call it, gives you the greatest ability to push food away and not care about it. It actually is joyful to realize when you are full and want no more food.

Two months after my surgery, I had the opportunity to "cat sit" for an American family in Paris. They were living in a beautiful apartment there and they wanted to vacation in the United States for the summer. I was able to see my daughter, Jennifer and my wonderful son-in-law, Philippe, who live in Paris and to immerse myself in French culture. Even though I had been in monthly phone contact with my surgeon's office, I didn't understand how to maximize the Golden Period and the important role protein played in how I healed from this surgery. In retrospect, I could have done more for my health if I had been more knowledgeable and aware. I could have understood my role better if I had been in contact with other patients from a support group that had an effective leader. Consequently, I ate a half of a cracker and a tiny sliver of cheese and thought I was nourishing myself. Although happy to be losing weight, I realize now that I didn't nourish myself well and, as a result, I could hardly concentrate.

As you heal from surgery, recognize that your body has gone through an enormous process and that it deserves rest, good nutrition, exercise and healthy thought. The wisdom of those who have gone before you is invaluable.

Your New Stomach

Now you are learning about your new stomach. It helps to visualize a chamois cloth. When a wet chamois dries, it becomes hard and not too pliable.[14] Similarly, your new stomach pouch has been fashioned from a part of the stomach that is the least distensible, and it is also swollen and irritable from the surgery.

For a while after surgery, placing food in your pouch is an unusual experience. Unlike before surgery, now your body will tell you *early* in your meal when you have put enough food in your pouch. The food you have eaten mixes with mucous in your pouch and swells to some degree, thus giving you a feeling of fullness quite early in the meal. This awareness may be a new sensation since eating prior to surgery was fairly unconscious. When you feel *satisfied*, not necessarily *full*, stop eating! *That's the gift of the surgery! Early satiety.*

One saying goes, "When you are full, your plate is empty." Let your saying be, "When I am *satisfied*, my plate is empty."

Behavioral Changes

At times, forgetting that your new stomach is restrictive, you may overeat and feel a sticking sensation, or some other discomfort, or you may vomit the food. Occasional vomiting indicates you are eating food improperly – *either the wrong food, too much food, the wrong consistency of a food, or eating too fast.* Use an occasional vomiting episode as a learning tool to modify your eating habits.

Gastric juices, produced in the large portion of the stomach, do not enter the little pouch, but mix farther down the digestive tract in the intestines. Since there is no gastric acid in the pouch now, vomiting means that the last food ingested "rolls out" *without* the bitter, acidic aftertaste of gastric reflux. In fact, gastric bypass surgery is sometimes used to cure Gastroesophageal Reflux Disease. (GERD)

In these early post-operative months, try eating untested foods at home instead of in a restaurant. If the need to vomit arises, you are not going to suddenly have to do it at the restaurant table, however, you may feel uncomfortable and need to seek out the closest restroom to relieve your discomfort. The privacy of home is probably preferable.

Here are some small behavioral changes that can net you a large result in your success:

➤ Eat from a small saucer instead of a big dinner plate. The food will look more plentiful. Did you ever wonder why salad plates were invented? They are really for gastric bypass patients to be used as dinner plates!

➤ Place a *small* bite of food in your mouth. Chew *slowly* and *thoroughly*.

➤ Eat with a baby spoon or with chopsticks, whatever will slow you down. Put down eating utensils after each bite.

➤ Don't serve food family style by placing large platters of food on the table. It encourages eating bigger portions and taking second helpings. Family style serving sets the stage for returning to bulk eating when there is a doubling in the size of your pouch six months after your operation.

➤ *Between* meals "load up" on water. You are more likely *thirsty* than hungry and don't know it.

➤ Throw away the food remaining on your plate! Despite what our mothers told us, nobody in China or anywhere else for that matter, ever profited from our being members of the Clean Plate Club.

It feels good when food does not have power over you.

As a society, generally, we eat too much and too fast. Look at the restaurant portions we are served. They are even called "Supersize," "King Size", "Great Biggie". We are accustomed to eating on the run, standing at the counter, or wolfing down food in the car. The rapid consumption of food will no longer feel good to you as you might experience a sticking sensation.

So, sit down at a table to eat quality food. Eat slowly. Sense your food. Stop eating when you feel satisfied. Toss out extra food at meal's end. Consider yourself a more "dainty" eater now. Again, get used to tossing food away. It's a liberating exercise.

Note: During this period of getting to know your new anatomy, a food that feels uncomfortable today, often feels just fine in a week or two as your pouch heals and becomes less irritable. Be patient.

The consistency of the food you eat makes a big difference. If you eat a piece of dry chicken breast, for instance, and it feels as if it "sticks", try preparing it in chicken broth so that it soaks up the moisture of the broth and is softer and more comfortable in your pouch. If the sticking continues, however, drink a mixture of a *little* water with a pinch of unseasoned meat tenderizer dissolved in it. That should help to break down the food. Try the offending food again later in your recovery.

During my Golden Period, vegetarian refried beans became one of my best choices. I also made my own lentil soup into which I added silken tofu, beans, chicken or a beaten egg. That was one high protein mixture! If I were only going to get a little food in, I wanted it to be the most concentrated nutrition I could create.

Often I added fresh, seasonal vegetables like zucchini and overcooked them a little so they were soft. They lost some of the vitamins by overcooking them, but at least I could eat them again. So experiment with high quality, nutritious foods and vary their preparation.

Each day will be a little different with your food experience. If you vomit a meal, as an example, your stomach may feel a little tender the next time you eat. Remember you can always "go backwards," so to speak, for a meal or two. For instance, if the skins on the beans in a bean soup don't feel comfortable to you, throw the soup into the blender. This way you will get a high protein mixture of a consistency that feels good in your stomach.

Weigh Yourself Daily

Some people advocate not weighing daily, but I disagree. The purpose is not to place emphasis on the scale, the "Iron Goddess of Weight Loss", but, instead, to *de-emphasize* the scale. Hopefully, since it is only *one measurement* of weight loss, you will learn not to have an ecstatic, dance-on-your-tippy-toes day if you lose weight, nor a day of depression if you don't. It is just information at a point in time. That's all. Within a year or so your weight should be where you want it to be, so why despair at each and every little bump along the way?

I weighed daily and I kept a weight graph (See Appendix). It was fun to see my weight trend down so consistently. I felt masterful and successful. The graph is also a teaching tool showing variances within any given month. You learn there are cycles to your weight loss and that a temporary slowdown is not a failure.

For instance, many women lose less weight the week prior to their menstrual period and more the week of and the week after. I noticed in my own Golden Period weight loss, at times, that if I had had a significant drop one day, the next day might show either no loss or slight gain as if my body wanted to find equilibrium. The body thinks it is starving. It doesn't recognize you would like to fit into a small pair of white jeans. When you can see a whole month demonstrated on a weight graph, you come to know and to anticipate your own weight loss pattern. Then, putting each month's chart end to end, helps you see how weight is lost in an uneven fashion. It is just the process of how the body burns its fat.

Exercising and building muscle also has a bearing on what the scale shows each day, as muscle tissue is heavier than fat. Other factors are your salt intake, stress level, water intake and just plain when your body is ready to let go of weight, the great unknown. Each day, you gain emotional investment in what has already been done. For instance, if you have just had a good exercise session at the gym, you will be less likely to want to "ruin it" by overeating. This emotional stake in your progress connects you with your body and becomes even more motivating as more and more weight comes off. Follow your program guidelines, that is, *protein first, vegetable, fruit, water, exercise and no snacking.* Allow yourself to do your very best during this period for optimum reward in your health, on the scale and in the fit of your clothes.

Constipation

Many people have a fear of having diarrhea after surgery since the old Jejuno-Ileal bypass carried that inevitability. Sometimes, the opposite is true. Constipation can be a problem when there is a diminished food intake. Here are some suggestions for dealing with constipation:

- Drink plenty of water *between* meals. Build up to 64 oz. a day, if you can.

- Exercise daily.

- Eat vegetables and fruit, as they are bulk forming.

- Sprinkle wheat germ on your food each day. (About a teaspoon) This is bulk forming, natural and tastes fine. (This may be uncomfortable early after the surgery.)

- If you are having a bout of constipation, some doctors suggest taking 2,000 to 4,000 mgs. Vitamin C a day for a few days, until your stool is normal.

- Avoid stimulant laxatives since they tend to cause a dependence on them. A stool softener is gentler than stimulant laxatives as a last resort.

Record Your Milestones In a Journal

During my weight loss phase, I went to the mall one day and tried on a dress in a size large in a store for "normal people." I didn't really expect it to fit but to my surprise and joy, it did! I hurried home and cut up my credit card from a store for plus sizes. I had been restricted to shopping there exclusively due to my weight. In an envelope and without any explanation, I mailed the many pieces to my daughter. She called me a few days later to tell me she understood the message and the freedom I felt. Now she peruses my closet to see what items I have purchased since her last visit that "might look better on her", as she says with a wink.

It makes it a meaningful journal if you write down your *milestones* along the way. It chronicles your remarkable progress much like a family baby book does. This is your rebirth, isn't it?

When did you first:

- Tie your shoe on the top and not on the side?

- Fit in the bathtub?

- Seat yourself without worrying that you would break the chair?

- Didn't feel the need to unzip your pants to be comfortable?

- Didn't have to lie down on a bed to get them zipped in the first place?

- Notice there is room to spare on the chair?

- Didn't drop food on your chest while you ate?

- Weren't embarrassed by stress incontinence?

- Felt comfortable you wouldn't bump into the glass in the shower?

- Were able to discontinue use of medications for high blood pressure, diabetes, high cholesterol, etc.

- Walked without pain?

- Climbed stairs and breathed easily?

- Didn't sweat heavily with minimum exertion?

- Wore a bathing suit?

- Crossed your legs?

- Shopped for clothes that had style and that you actually liked?

- Didn't have heartburn?

- Looked forward to meeting new people?

- Got a job promotion?

- Wore pants with a sewn-in waistband instead of elastic?

- Ran on the beach?

- Played softball with your children in the park?

- Rode an amusement park ride?

- Stood up for yourself?

- Chose an activity solely on the basis of whether it would be fun?

- Fit in a restaurant booth?

- Walked without getting shin splints?

- Took off your clothes in front of your mate without embarrassment?

- Danced in the rain?

- Wore jeans?

- Made love?

- Felt comfortable in your skin?

Revel in these milestones in your life because as adults we no longer have a report card to measure our successes. So give yourself your own report card by recording these milestones. They are the signs that you are taking your life back!

Save Some Old Clothes

I suggest saving one or two pieces of clothing from your top weight. At first you might not want to be reminded of how big they are, but later you will come to see them as a marker of where you started and as a measure of where you have gone. It is a visual reminder of your considerable progress.

Your weight changes rapidly in this Golden Period. Exchanging clothes in your support group or at a thrift shop will allow you to have "new" clothes as you reduce.

Regarding thrift stores, it is really amazing what people decide they no longer want to wear. Some people wear an article of clothing a few times in a season and then get rid of it when the weather changes. Those clothes are new enough for me! I have found treasures in thrift shops. I own a new 100% Cashmere jacket that I bought for $8 dollars. I found one store that received overbuys from a major department store. They had the tags still on them and I found suits for $5 to $10!

Feel free to donate the remainder of your larger clothes to someone behind you on the weight loss path. You do not need them anymore because you are through with dieting and weight cycling. You now know how to eat so that you are living at a healthy weight. You are elegant, calm, self-assured and surgically gifted! Take a breath of your new life.

ACTION LIST:

➢ Make a promise to yourself. Seriously now, raise your right hand and say, "I, _____(your name)_____, solemnly swear, never to consider myself on a diet again, but rather, I promise to eat in such a manner where I nourish my wonderful body, so help me _____."

➢ Become acquainted with your new stomach. Eat slowly sensing satiety.

➢ Chart your weight daily.

➢ Journal your progress and your milestones.

➢ Save some old clothes and pass the rest along.

8

Six Months and Beyond:
When Hunger Returns

My doctor told me to stop having intimate dinners for four. Unless there are three other people.

– Orson Welles

Never eat more than you can lift.

– Miss Piggy

Around Month 6, your hunger returns.

The gastric bypass is a wonderful aid, but a word of caution is in order. *It is not a panacea. It is a tool.* It makes lifestyle changes much, much easier than in the days of dieting, but you must understand that you can defeat this surgery and gain the weight back. If you ignore the body's signals and eat large portions, eat high carbohydrates foods, snack, graze and drink caloric beverages, you will be on your way to obesity again.

Your pouch is now a little less irritable and more distensible. The pouch doubles in size by six months, although it will still hold only around three to six ounces compared to the two quarts it held in your pre-surgical days. Initially, your pouch was about the size of your thumb and its knuckle. Now, as it increases in size, you will notice that you are able to eat more quantity and this is very frightening to most of us. What will you do when the hunger returns?

After five years, my own hunger hasn't returned to anything like the ravenous, "Let me eat the entire cow" level of my pre-surgical days. But I know that when I first felt even slight hunger, I worried with such thoughts as, "This surgery isn't working

anymore. I'm going to fail at this and gain all my weight back.
My pouch has gotten too big."

To minimize hunger, I eat so as not to become too hungry. And
that is what I would like to teach you to do.

I have heard people in my support groups say they first measure
their food and then try to put that amount into their pouch. In
other words, if their pouch is supposed to hold two ounces, they
measure out two ounces to consume. No more measuring! That's
"diet head thinking". It is now time for sensing and feeling what
goes into your stomach.

You will notice that after surgery, your pouch fluctuates in its
ability to accommodate food at any given time. It will not
necessarily respond to holding the same amount of food at each
meal. This is surprising to many of us since we are used to having
our stomachs allow for huge quantities of food at each sitting.

So –

- If you have a heavy protein serving at one meal, you may
  find that less food is accepted in the pouch at the next
  meal and that you are less hungry.

- If you have had an episode of vomiting, your pouch may
  be sore and it will not allow much food in it the next
  meal.

- If you are emotionally upset, food may feel unwelcome.

- If you have just had liquids, there may not be much room
  for solids to fit.

Again, this process involves mindfulness as to the comfort of your pouch. Sense the food as you eat. *Stop eating if you feel fullness or discomfort.* Eat with elegance.

If you disregard your body's signals, you will find that you overfill your pouch resulting in discomfort and possibly you will vomit.

The Most Important Advice In This Book

This advice applies *always and forever* after your surgery.

To avoid getting too hungry, eat this way:

➤ *Eat three meals each day, no more than five hours apart.*

➤ *Protein first. (about 2/3 of your meal).*(meat, fish, chicken, beans, etc.)

Protein suppresses your appetite and is crucial for rebuilding cells.

➤ *Eat a vegetable next.*

➤ *Then some fruit, not necessarily a whole one.*

Carbohydrates make you hungrier. Get your carbohydrates from vegetables and fruit, if possible. This eliminates refined and often nutritionally empty calories. Vegetables are an excellent source of vitamins A, C and folate. In addition, they provide minerals, including iron and magnesium. Vegetables are also naturally low in dietary fat.

Fruits are naturally low in sodium and they are an excellent source of fiber and carbohydrate. They provide generous amounts of vitamin A and C and potassium.

Rice, bread, tortillas, pasta and potatoes often swell in the pouch. I have found that since I become uncomfortable eating them, I have actually lost much of my taste for them.

➢ *No snacking.*

➢ *Drink 64 ounces of water a day.*

When you are depleted of water you can feel lethargic and dizzy. As this worsens, muscular endurance can diminish, concentration becomes difficult, and you become drowsy, impatient and headachy.

➢ *Exercise.*

Exercise

Before you wrinkle your nose at the idea of moving your body, let me make a few suggestions:

Exercise in a way that is consistent with your personality. Do what is fun for you. I choose to walk instead of bike ride, for instance, because the pace suits me. I love nature. I enjoy seeing how the flowers change on my route day by day. I also go nuts for dogs. They give me comic relief every time I see them. I am getting fresh air and exercise as I go and I have *fun*.

On one such walk I encountered a gray, standard poodle and I proceeded to discuss life with him. Finally, I realized that a human must be at the other end of the leash. I looked up, and to my surprise, there was Jack Lemmon. Although Mr. Lemmon was patient, the dog and I were far more pleased with the encounter than he was.

You see, moving your body can consist of an organized sport, a structured plan, or just something active that allows you to move in a joyful way. What is joyful for you?

Try to consciously add steps to your day. Climb a flight of stairs. Park your car across a parking lot, break into dance, play ball with your children.

Exercise in a way that is opposite to your personality. For instance, if you have a Type-A personality, are rushing through your life, try a Yoga class. It will feel uncomfortable. It's OK to feel uncomfortable. Yoga will force you to slow down, to empty your mind. It will challenge your brain. It's like running forward and all of a sudden changing direction to run backwards for a while. It feels odd but it stimulates you.

If you tend to be introverted and quiet, try your hand at racquetball or tennis, for example. Fast-paced sports that require interaction with an opponent, quick reflexes and mental alertness, stimulate you, as well.

Look to the athletes of different sports. What characteristics of their bodies would you like to acquire for your own? For instance, swimmers tend to have broad shoulders and strong, slender, beautifully shaped legs. That sport will develop your body in a similar way.

Nutritional Supplements

"Because certain elements are absorbed in only a single area of the small intestine (such as Vitamin B-12 in the lowermost portion of the ileum, iron primarily in the duodenum and folic acid in the upper jejunum), surgical removal results in deficiency".[4]

The bottom part of the stomach, that part which has been severed from the pouch, produces a protein called *Intrinsic Factor*. This protein helps the body absorb Vitamin B-12, an essential vitamin for health. Since this portion of the stomach has been bypassed, our bodies cannot absorb Vitamin B-12 by swallowing it in tablet form.

Over time, the body will suffer neurological problems without Vitamin B-12, very much like multiple sclerosis, sometimes to an irreparable degree. *It is imperative, therefore, to replace this important vitamin regularly in a way the body can absorb it.* Special *sublingual* Vitamin B-12 tablets for use under the tongue are readily available and inexpensive. Another way is to have your doctor inject it once a month.

Note. *Avoid* taking medications in *tablet form*, whenever possible. It is preferable to ingest all medications, other then the Vitamin B-12, in either a capsule, chewable, gelcap, or liquid form. Many times, hard tablets, especially large ones, simply pass through the gastrointestinal tract without sufficient breakdown to be absorbed and are, therefore, of little if any nutritional or medicinal value.

Calcium also should be supplemented. *Calcium Citrate* is the preparation most easily digested by bariatric patients, not Calcium Carbonate.

Take these vitamin and mineral supplements *daily*:

- Calcium (preferably, *Calcium Citrate*)

- Multivitamins and

- Vitamin B-12.

There is controversy regarding the necessity for supplementing *Iron*. Check with your doctor.

No snacking between meals. I am surprised at how little true hunger I feel. Never having allowed myself to get hungry in the past, it astounded me to learn that if I just let myself feel the hunger for a while it would pass in a few minutes and death would not ensue! It just disappeared. If you *must* take food in between meals, rarely and for damage control, make sure it is a small amount of *protein.* A few bites of chicken will stave off your hunger, if indeed it is hunger and not thirst.

Did you know most obese people do not differentiate between hunger and thirst? So if you drink some water first you might be amazed that you feel full and that you weren't hungry at all.

These are the guidelines and that's it! No "diet head." No feelings of deprivation.

Protein Foods

The importance of proteins cannot be overemphasized. I am not advocating enormous amounts of this food source, rather simply explaining the benefits of protein.

Protein assists in the maintenance of lean muscle mass. Without adequate protein, our bodies will favor burning muscle tissue in place of fat. We may burn lean muscle from anywhere the body can find it. As stated, it also helps you feel full longer after a meal. Protein is important for wound healing and for hair growth. *Without adequate protein, hair loss during the period of rapid weight loss, usually between the third and sixth month, can be upsetting.* And it does grow back as you eat more protein foods.

Your goal is to eat about 60 to 80 grams of protein a day, depending on whether you are male or female.

Here is a list of foods and the protein grams per average serving they provide:

Anchovies	6		Humus	4
Bacon	6		Lamb	29
Bass	19		Liver	23
Beans	6-8		Lobster	15
Beef	16-21		Milk	8
Broccoli	3		Oysters	10
Cheese	14		Peas	4
Chicken	35		Pork roast	15
Clams	6		Rabbit	25
Cottage cheese	13		Salmon	22
Crab	16-17		Sardines	6
Duck	26		Shrimp	4-5
Egg	5		Soy milk	7
Ham	14-15		Spinach	3

Swordfish	22		Turkey	25
Tofu	20		Veal	31
Tuna	23		Yogurt	6

A caution when reading the supermarket label on the food item: the quoted protein amounts may be based on serving sizes too large for you, so the amount of protein may be misleading.

Gastric Bypass Surgery Benefits

You may already be discovering the benefits of this remarkable surgery:

- Less obsession/compulsion in regard to food.

- No calorie counting.

- A variety of choices.

- A way to restrict the amount eaten.

- A way to have early satiety.

- A way to feel "normal".

- A feeling of abundance.

- A way of eating to be healthy for life.

ACTION LIST:

➢ Drink 64 ounces of water a day.

➢ One-half hour before the next meal, stop drinking.

➢ Eat only three meals each day, no more than five hours apart.

  ▪ Protein first. (about 2/3 of your meal)

  ▪ A vegetable next.

  ▪ Then, some fruit.

➢ One-half hour after eating, begin to sip water and continue to water load.

➢ Obtain your carbohydrates from vegetables and fruit.

➢ Take Vitamin B-12, Multivitamins and Calcium Citrate daily.

➢ No snacking between meals.

➢ Exercise in a way consistent with your personality.

➢ Exercise in a way opposite to your personality.

➢ Smile and laugh a lot.

9

Overcoming Self-Defeat
and Subterfuge

"You, yourself, as much as anybody in the universe, deserve your love and affection."

– *Buddha*

Feelings of Deprivation

My belief is that feelings of deprivation eventually lead to bingeing. To think that with your new anatomy you are deprived and that delicious, nutritious, high quality food is for others and not for you, is a fallacy. In fact, you deserve the very best food, clothes, etc. that your money can buy. And that goes for your choices of friends and associates and jobs, too. Self-esteem is crucial to creating a healthy new you, a new mentality along with a new body. Give yourself the best you possibly can. The more you feel rewards in other areas of your life, the less you'll feel a need to binge.

Self-Defeat And Subterfuge

The truth is that I feel "normal" for the first time in my life. I obsess much less over food. I fill up quickly and I am satisfied. I rarely experience the "I gotta have that" feeling. It is natural at this time to feel oneself as being "bullet proof." But my program is not bullet proof. It needs to be worked with a focused eye each and every day.

I know of one woman who defeated her program by planning to purposely "dump" on her days off from work. She bought large bags of candy, locked herself in her bedroom and ate until she was sick and fell asleep. She spent all that money for surgery. All the hope, pain and effort were for nothing, it seems, as she is now regaining her weight.

Another woman called me at the office crying that she had regained 75 pounds. Why did she wait so long to get help? I wished she had called me earlier.

If my weight goes up more than a couple of pounds, I concentrate on eating mostly dense proteins, such as, a small steak that day. No big sacrifice, right? It sits heavily in my stomach and it gives me satiety for hours. I also don't eat many carbohydrates that day. If my weight corrects the next day, I can relax more. The obvious point is that it is far easier to work with two pounds of weight gain than with 75 pounds gained. *If you never allow more than a two-pound fluctuation, it will be easy to maintain the weight you have lost.*

The woman that had delayed seeking help had a complete collapse of her weight loss program. Long before that happens, lapses occur. All day, everyday, we are faced with lifestyle decisions. There is a constant fork in the road. We can either go to the gym with a friend, or we can decide to view rental movies sitting on the couch. We can either drink water, as recommended, or we can grab a can of soda. We can plan a social gathering at a restaurant, or we can plan a hike through a forest. These decisions point us in a direction towards health and a mobile body, or away from them. The accumulations of many small decisions are like little pearls strung together to make a necklace. If you add one good decision to another good decision to another and so on, day by day, you are rewarded on the scale. So, just eat as advised and exercise. Weight loss is just calories "in" and calories "out" and the big picture takes care of itself. You *will* accomplish your weight loss.

Nonetheless, as humans, each of us has an occasional lapse. In an effort to divert ourselves from the obsessions of food, we put time and distance between our emotions and recreational eating, but still, we chose to eat. There is nothing to be gained by self-recrimination.

It creates shame and the resultant desire to assuage that pain with food. Shame begins the downward spiral into eating to salve our hurt feelings.

Resume immediately all the practical tools you know give you health. You have an arsenal of new behaviors and activities from which to pick. Soon you will be back on track.

A total collapse, as with the woman who phoned me despairingly, is another story. That kind of destruction of our new program of healthful living, robs us of self-esteem and engenders fear. It takes effort to correct the situation. Again, continue to take many small steps in the right direction. Here are some suggestions:

- Call your surgeon and make an appointment to "face the music." The reality of seeing your weight gain written in black and white in his office, breaks the pattern of avoidance. Then compliment yourself on your courage. Hopefully, your surgeon is a compassionate and wise practitioner and you will be able to say to him, "I am having trouble with my program, but I am committed to getting back on track again."

- Encourage your doctor and the staff to be your cheerleaders. With their encouragement, you will have that "new start" feeling and be motivated again when you walk out the door.

- There is a movement in Tai Chi, a Chinese system of physical exercises designed for self-defense and meditation, called Face the Tiger. To Face the Tiger is to face your fears. I keep a small Chinese bottle with a picture of a tiger on it on my desk as a continual reminder to face my fears.

- Call a friend to make an appointment to meet for a walk. I show up when I make appointments with others, whereas I won't always keep that promise to myself.

- Use your support group for that same purpose. Many times the facilitator will have a program planned for the evening. I always do. But when someone raises her hand and asks a question of concern about her health, I relax the agenda and I follow in the direction the group needs to go. Don't be shy about asking for help in support groups. It shows that you have the self-esteem to get your needs met. Also, consider the fact that everyone learns from everyone else. A person who was too shy to raise her hand might be eternally grateful that you have come forward.

- Exercise. You are able to do more now and it is easier. Did you know that exercise elevates your mood? Did you know that exercise burns consumed calories? Did you know you are more likely to drop weight the next day if you exercise? Of course you knew these facts. But did you know that exercising *prevents* the formation of new fat cells? Yes, indeed! That's a great mental image as you walk along, isn't it? Instead of sitting at home because you overate a bit and sabotaging your efforts further, exercise and *prevent fat cell formation!*

Find A Good Support Group

Support Groups range from the purely social to the most structured in nature. But, unfortunately, my experience shows that, as a rule, the format decided by the facilitator of the group leaves the members with little say about the process.

I have attended groups where people were mumbling angrily about the facilitator's chosen lecture topic that evening while walking through the door. *The support group belongs to you!* Ideally, a support group is:

- A forum in which you will learn from the experience of others.

- A place to lend your experience and hope.

- A place to gain skills for living in the world during and after weight loss.

- A place to practice socialization skills.

- A place to safely reveal your vulnerabilities.

- A place to laugh and to cry.

- A place to give service to others.

If your support group is constructed mainly to provide information for investigating *pre-operative* individuals, ask your surgeon to create another group specifically oriented to the needs of *post-operative* patients. If unsuccessful, then start your own group and find a leader who is well versed in the *behavioral* aspects of weight issues.

Creating A Fully Functioning Support Group

Here are some ideas to create a more fully functioning support group:

- Create an "Angel" System. This is a system whereby the group designates volunteers, or "Angels" to visit new gastric bypass patients in the hospital to give encouragement and hope. It is frightening to feel that we are alone in our problem. Note, however, it is not within the scope of their role to give medical advice of any kind, nor to launch into their own "war stories." The Angels from your group lend a sympathetic ear and just listen. We all feel better when someone expresses, "Yes, I went through that too, but it all turned out well."

  Create a calendar that designates who will be the Angel each day. Set guidelines for what constitutes an "appropriate visit." Allow the patient to leave a sign on the hospital door if she would prefer not to have a visitor that day.

  Angels may exchange phone numbers with new patients. The patient now has a "lifeline connection" to someone outside of the hospital when she has a need to talk to a fellow traveler, who understands what it feels like to undergo gastric bypass surgery.

- Create a large notebook/journal of testimonials written by your members for new investigators of the surgery to read. These new people gain comfort and hope from your successes. Remember they still suffer. They have come to get the kind of support they can't find anywhere else.

They need your wisdom now. Bring the notebook/journal to each meeting.

- Confidentiality is an ever-present requirement in the medical profession. Doctors must keep your name and other information private. Therefore, have your group take the responsibility of creating an e-mail/phone system network of willing members and designate a member to be the keeper of these addresses and phone numbers. That roster becomes the communications network for the group, enabling members to call another member if they are having a difficult moment with food.

- Suggest to your group facilitator names of prospective speakers you think will enhance your group's interests. These speakers will help keep information fresh and interesting.

- Create a journal/notebook that informs and gives hope to the *supporters* of the surgical weight loss patients. As these friends and loved ones come to group to learn about helping in the surgical weight loss process, they can write their own concerns in the journal and read the concerns of others who came before them. These loved ones and friends are our backbone and strength during our time of rapid change. More than anyone else, they stand to lose the most if you are ill or if they lose you. They worry about us so we need to offer them our support, also. Then, after you have had your surgery and are doing well, your supporter can come back to the journal to add her own encouraging thoughts and feelings from her new perspective.

- Create an activities program for members. Designate a member to research which gyms have group rates or specials in your community. See if there is a gym that will create a class for only overweight people. It is so much more comfortable to exercise with people working toward the same goal. The recreational leader can also research different events in the community such as a "walk" for your group as a fundraiser. Organize specialty exercise groups such as a Walking Club, Meet At The Treadmill Group, Dance Group, Meet For A Beach Stroll Group, Basketball At The Y Group, Softball Team, etc.

- Have a committee seek out service businesses in the community offering member discounts, such as hair styling, facials, massages, etc.

- Create a group cookbook of foods appropriate for gastric bypass patients. Chapters can be divided into Immediately After Surgery, The Golden Period, When the Hunger Returns, etc.

- Create a social network with whom to attend events. It's fun to go places as a group and easier to venture out. There may be discounts available on group ticket purchases.

- Plan a holiday party that serves *only* healthy foods. It's a relief to emerge from a holiday thinner and without guilt.

- Assign a *short time* in each meeting for a patient testimonial. It offers strength and hope to others to hear how we have faced our fears and triumphed.

- Create a way for your group to "give back." Is there a fellow member who needs the group's support for their children at Christmas? Is there a community project that would increase awareness of the suffering of people of size? Can you sponsor an event during the holidays that is not food-oriented to give members, who are alone, a loving place to celebrate?

- Create a group photo album with a page devoted to each member that includes a "before" picture, some photos on the way down and a picture at goal. The album offers inspiration to the newcomers and raises the self-esteem of the members.

- Create a clothing exchange so that clothes can be recycled. It benefits the giver and the recipient alike.

- Ask if there are members who would be willing to stand at the back of the room after the meeting to answer questions and offer their hope to the investigators of surgery and to their supporters. Extend the welcoming hand of your group.

- Your support group will function more independently if it has a financial base. A treasury allows the group to hire special speakers, fund special events and to allow self-direction. Create ways for your group to earn money. (A bake sale is out though!)

ACTION LIST:

➢ Allot time after your support group meeting to encourage socialization. Arrange an after-support-group meeting with other members of your support group.

➢ Organize two activities from the chapter list or two items of your own choosing.

[10]

Moving Through Space

"The game isn't over 'til it's over."

– Yogi Berra

Exercise is an essential component of your long-term weight loss success. Here are some thoughts about moving your body through space and the ways I found to make it fun. I am not an exercise physiologist nor would I presume to profess to be an expert on exercise. Thousands of books have been written on the topic. Instead, it is your *attitude* toward exercise that I am addressing.

I once asked a psychologist what he thought was the number one reason why people are overweight. Without hesitation, he answered, "Fossil fuels." He was in the habit of riding his bike 14 miles to work.

As I lost weight, I exercised more and more. I started with a small amount of walking. As my weight decreased, I walked faster and farther partly because of the reward on the scale the next day, and, partly because it gave me such pleasure to know I could move so much more easily. I wanted to do what obesity had prevented me from doing in the past. I walked if it rained. I walked if it snowed. I walked in hot summers. I walked because I found my ability to move joyful.

At one point in my weight loss, my friend, Laura, suggested we take up racquetball even though we were still well over 200 pounds. I weighed 230 pounds actually, and I doubted my ankles were going to hold me up for such a venture. Despite my misgivings, we bought equipment, took lessons and learned to play the sport. I'm sure, in retrospect, we were quite a sight on the courts!

There was no way we were going to take the sport as seriously as the men around us and so when Laura and I played, we would bet all kinds of "rewards" on each point.

"OK, for the chateau in France," she would say, "let's play this point." I would counter with other luxuries, such as, a new Rolls Royce, or a villa in Italy. Each time she won a point, she would yell out, "And the crowd went wild!" and hold up two fingers in a "V." She then would make her "crowd-went-wild war yelp" and we would dissolve into laughter that sometimes left us seated on the court floor.

Who cared who won, really? We exercised. We had fun. We laughed. We sat down.

Likewise, I discovered the fun of playing water volleyball with other overweight people. After the first couple of moments of checking each other out, we really didn't notice each other's weight. The water made us buoyant and our competitive spirits took over. We were learning to structure our time so that we were moving our bodies and not devoting our evenings to watching television. The swimming pool became an inviting place to exercise at the end of the day, soothing our sore feet and aching joints.

On many occasions my friend, Bob and I would spend the evening in the indoor pool. As we walked in circles in the water, we sang all the songs we could remember. You have never heard anything until you have heard Bob sing *Amazing Grace* at the top of his lungs over waves of water in a pool. What he lacked in formal training, he made up for in enthusiasm and sheer volume.

Finally, I got to the point where I was receiving invitations to date. On one such occasion, I was asked out to a dance club. I accepted, dressed up and looked forward to my evening. When I got onto the dance floor with my date, to my horror I realized there were many dances I had never learned. I resolved to find a way to learn to dance them.

The next day, I recounted my embarrassment to my friend, Joe. He told me not to worry, that he would have a solution for me by dinnertime. That evening, true to his word, Joe told me to be ready on Friday night for a surprise. He had generously spent his afternoon researching places to dance that had a "nice crowd." On Friday, he took me to a country western dance club. The men there had old-fashioned manners and took dancing seriously. I watched for a long time. I loved the country western dances and I ached to get in on the fun. As I gazed around the room, I saw a man who danced like a "Country Western Baryshnikov." I really wanted to dance with him.

I watched him for a long time, feeling queasy at the thought of asking him to dance and the possibility of his rejection. Many women wanted to dance with him and breaking into that circle seemed daunting. Finally, with every ounce of courage that I could muster, I slowly crossed a "mile-long" dance floor. Introducing myself, I told him I didn't know how to do the different dances but that if he would teach me, I would go home and practice in my living room until I could do them well.

I told Mike about my weight loss efforts and he responded by revealing to me that even though he was slender, he took up dancing as a form of exercise because his doctor said it would lower his cholesterol level. He then very sweetly adopted me for the evening, teaching me the Texas Two-Step. Dear Mike proved to be a kind and patient instructor. I did learn to dance and soon

Mike was calling me each weekend to make sure I showed up. We were each other's only dance partners and we danced every dance together until closing. We ended up being dance partners for years, dancing three nights a week. Mike lowered his cholesterol and I lost my weight.

Near my home at that time was a hotel that had a dance lounge catering to the obese crowd. We teasingly called it the Crisco Disco. Imagine an entire club devoted only to overweight people! We got a chance to practice dancing and some social skills with "our own." We were in a safe haven. It was a great advantage to be "exercising" with other obese people, who had similar goals, particularly when the concept of attending a health club was too overwhelming. There were too many skinny twenty-year olds teaching classes there for my comfort. What did they know about my overweight body and aging joints, I wondered.

As I progressed in my weight loss, I did a partial run and a partial power walk for one straight hour with my friend Marla each morning. I am only 5'5". Marla, on the other hand, is 5'10". In heels she could be scary! If I didn't push myself to keep up, Marla would lose me on the corners as we circled the mall. She was a perfect exercise partner for me as she presented a challenge to my program. When we did our power walk, the customers at the mall's McDonald's would cheer us on as we went by. We yelled playfully to them that they should get up and join us. "Hah", we laughed. "Let 'em catch us!"

One evening on a ship cruise, I watched as a very rotund African-American woman dressed in traditional African garb walked out on to the dance floor of the ship. Noticing her size, I held my breath as she kicked off her shoes and began to dance. She moved, however, with grace, joy in her dance and a broad smile on her face. People clapped to the music and cheered her on. I wanted to learn African dance, too, so I kicked off my shoes, walked up in back of her and followed her lead. I will just tell you my hips did things they had never been known to do before.

I have met many people who, after weight loss surgery, pursued the dreams they couldn't realize as chubby children. Some took up tap dance and ballet. Others tried sports for the first time. I met one woman who invented her own version of rollerblading using ski poles. She wore a gold helmet, blue kneepads and a red cape!

Most slender people have a form of exercise they learned as children that they can bring along into their adult lives. Many obese individuals do not. It's OK to reconstruct your childhood, don't you think? Remember all those activities you missed out on and give them a try. I have been rollerblading, roller-skating, played racquetball, went body surfing, long distance walking and hiking in the Andes. I have danced new dances, played volleyball and water volleyball, went power walking, jogging, water walking, ocean swimming and did Tai Chi. I still have many more to try. While I have no desire to jump out of an airplane, a kayak is definitely in my future.

One year, I joined a walking/running club. All the members started at the same time together but, once started, chose their own pace. I thought I was a whiz until, part of the way out, I looked up and there was 90-year old Sammy, running past me. He was lean and lanky, with a red sweatband around a few gray hairs. When I arrived at the designated watering hole, he had his water in hand and was sitting there smiling.

Why am I telling you these stories? Because people move towards what is pleasurable. If something makes you laugh, gives you joy and it is fun, you will be more likely to choose it to do again.

Remember, you don't have to be perfect or even be good at what you attempt. Relax your expectations of yourself and just *enjoy* the activity for the fun you derive.

Get a group of friends together who are also overweight and who have similar goals to yours and enjoy yourselves. Plan activities to move! Don't meet for lunch. Meet for a walk with your dogs on the beach. Don't go to a movie. Hike a trail and collect pinecones. If your activity is not fun, it is likely that sooner or later you will abandon your efforts. It is less important, in my opinion, if you hit your target heart zone for exactly 20-40 minutes *each* and *every* day, seven days a week and more important that you get fresh air, laugh, move a lot, and feel joy. I know the weight will come off if you push yourself to sweat. Imagine your doctor has written a prescription for you to go have fun!

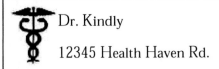 Dr. Kindly

12345 Health Haven Rd.

YOUR NAME HERE

RX: **HAVE FUN EACH AND EVERY DAY**.

Massage

While you are having fun, how about a massage? Massage gives you the opportunity to connect with your finite body as you lose weight, that is, you gain a sense of where your body now ends.

It is also a place to feel different emotions and memories. I grieved more than once for people I had lost as I received a massage, letting my tears flow. My therapist created a safe haven for me to do so.

At one time, I devoted my own massage practice to overweight people so they could come to someone who would help them accept their bodies. They knew I had no prejudice, nor judgment about their large size. In fact I saw them as quite courageous to allow themselves to be that vulnerable. I felt honored that they chose me as their therapist.

Never Too Old To Start

Even if you have been tied to the couch all your life, it is possible to learn to enjoy movement.

Once Al, a man in his 70's, approached me. "I would like to take an exercise class but I have never done it before and I don't even have anything to wear for exercise." I assured Al that I was the Shopper Woman of All Time and to meet me later. We met and I drove him to the mall. He was thrilled that he could fit into a sweat suit.

As I passed the gym the next night, I glanced in the window. There was Al, who had joined an aerobics class. He was wearing a shocking red sweat suit and a matching sweatband around his grey hair. Most notable was the broad grin on his white-bearded face. What courage he had to embark on an exercise regimen late in his life and what a smiling spirit shone.

Exercise Commitment

Part of the formula to lose weight is to go with the winners. If you want a workout, look around for someone who is farther ahead in the weight loss process than you are and is serious about her program. Ask to exercise with her a few times a week. Your exercise mate then pulls you along to do more than you might attempt on your own.

The mall is a wonderful place to get a walking program going. It is protected from weather, well lighted, has security guards and bathrooms. You are stimulated by other people and by the changing window displays in the stores. Try tapes of music that keep a good walking cadence going for an hour. You can listen, sing and walk. My friend, Shelley and I have been known to break into dance for no apparent reason while walking and we have never been asked to leave a mall ... yet.

If you must spend an evening in front of the TV, don't just watch the stimulating food commercials. Place a set of weights by your chair. When the commercial comes on, do a set of arm exercises. See how virtuous you feel?

The emphasis on bodybuilding with overweight individuals initially is on the upper body. Usually women, left on their own, will choose lower body exercises. Most overweight people, however, already have developed strong muscles in their lower bodies. Often times, carrying around extra weight has built up their legs, but strengthening the upper body has been overlooked.

Increasing the muscle size raises the resting metabolic rate. This means you burn extra calories for a much longer time after exercising.

What's #1?

Structure your day by making a written agenda. Where did you place exercise? *If it is not #1, in all likelihood, it will fall to the bottom of your list and you will not do it.* There is a vast difference between intention and commitment. All the good intentions in the world won't get the job done. Soon you will fall out of the habit of putting on your walking shoes and getting out there if you do not place exercise as #1 on your list.

Make the opportunity to exercise easy for yourself. Leave a pair of walking shoes in the trunk of your car. If you find yourself in an area you might like to explore, you'll be ready. Also, there is a greater likelihood of exercising more if you leave the house wearing walking shoes than wearing dress shoes.

To illustrate an example of commitment, my friend, Susanne, vice president of a securities brokerage firm, awakens at 4:00 AM everyday so she can be at the gym by 5:00. She participates in a Masters Swimmers Program and she swims laps for speed for an hour each day. She then showers, dresses and goes to work. That's commitment!

On the average, it takes three weeks to adopt a new habit. So just get up each day and do it. Don't ask yourself if you want to. Don't ask yourself if you'd like to. Don't consult the weatherman. Don't search your horoscope or ask universal gods to guide you in your decision. Just mindlessly put on your shoes and get out there and move it!

One note of caution: many people tax their bodies in exercise and sports past moderation, without regard for their aging joints. They may run a marathon when their bodies are built for sprinting and are weekend warriors two days a week, couch potatoes the other five. Remember the story of *The Tortoise and the Hare?* Consistency of effort is the key.

Chinese philosophy teaches us moderation in all things including exercise. Tai Chi, for instance, respects the body's changing ability, calms the spirit and teaches one to go within oneself in meditation. It is practiced from childhood through advanced adulthood within the Chinese culture.

Yoga stretches the body, keeping it limber, and massages the organs through exercise.

Walk

Check with your doctor for his approval to begin an exercise program. Walking is a great place to start. It is easy. You *don't* have to walk fast or far. The only necessary expense is the purchase of good, comfortable, walking shoes. Go for function, not fashion! Look for the following:

- Shoes made specifically for walking or cross-trainers.

- Adequate toe room. (often your feet will swell as you walk)

- Snug heels.

- Flexibility.

- Firm arch supports.

- Well-cushioned impact points.

There is a guided imagery I invented for myself when I walk that I'd like to share with you. I envision two colors—one of a clear, brilliant blue sky, the other is a vast wheat field, with tall sheaves of beige wheat waving in the breeze. I am a scythe and as I walk, I cut a path through the wheat. Whoa! Does that ever feel powerful

to me! You can create your own visual image to empower yourself
as you walk.

Here are some of the benefits of walking:

- Fun.

- Part of a rehabilitation plan for heart patients.

- Lowers cholesterol.

- Encourages social contact.

- Aerates the lungs.

- Lowers blood pressure.

- Lowers diabetic's need for supplemental insulin.

- Gets you out into the sunshine converting Vitamin E.

- Relieves muscle tension.

- Relieves headaches.

- Lowers stress.

- Improves mood and gives a vibrant energy level.

- Gives you time to think.

- Is a barometer of how your body is performing each day.

- Increases metabolic rate. (the rate at which calories are burned).

- Burns fat and spares lean muscle.

- Tones and builds muscle.

- Reduces appetite.

- Helps prevent constipation.

- Hinders the formation of new fat cells.

- Gives a sense of mastery and competency and raises self-esteem.

- Stimulates the senses.

- Helps clear your mind.

- Increases bone strength.

- Attracts other people who are taking care of their health, too.

- Provides satisfaction of knowing you have done something positive for your body each day.

- Reduces the likelihood of developing gallstones.

- Enhances sleep.

- Increases alertness.

- Gives your body a beautiful contour.

- Makes you laugh and feel happy.

- Improves your reaction time and balance.

- Helps with sagging skin from weight loss.

- Helps weight maintenance.

- Increases supply of oxygen to cardiac muscle.

- Is inexpensive.

- Lowers risk of developing colon cancer.

- Lowers incidence of diverticular disease.

- Reduces joint swelling in arthritic individuals.

- Strengthens muscles to prevent falls and broken bones.

- Lowers the incidence of prostatic hyperplasia in men.

- Stimulates your Pineal Gland. (look it up)

- Accelerates weight loss.

- Provides increased opportunities for socializing.

- Improves gait and balance.

- Builds muscle that burns calories more efficiently.

- Can increase bone density.

- Improves muscle strength.

- Allows you to meet a great dog along the way. (Very important!)

That's a *considerable* amount of benefit from only one activity.

One day I was walking around Balboa Island, California. Its houses are built in a circle around the island with a walking path between them and the ocean. I had been curious about seeing the beautiful houses on the island although I had never been in one of them. On my walk, I encountered an elderly woman coming out of her house and I complimented her on the tile work on her patio. She explained to me that she and her husband, who had died recently, had designed the entire house many years ago and they had lived there since early in their marriage. I told her how much I enjoy walking on the strand and seeing the beautiful houses.

She turned to me and asked, "Why don't you just come in and I'll tell you all about my house?" I took her up on her invitation, enjoyed her stories and the architecture of her home and had a delightful time. I waved to her each day after that when on my walk.

Take a CD or tape player along to give yourself a musical lift and to keep a rhythm as you walk. The music energizes you.

Dress in layers so you can remove them as you heat up.

Walk in such a way that you vary your length of stride and swing your arms, especially above the level of your heart. This will increase your heart rate and the intensity of your workout if your heart rate drops. I find strangers avoid me when I do this, however.

When we connect with our bodies, exercise offers a barometer of how our body is feeling that day. Some days we tire more quickly and some days we have more energy. If you had an alcoholic drink the night before, you will find it affects your performance negatively the next day. Progressively, you will get in touch with the status of your body. For most of us who haven't been involved with exercise, it now becomes a revelation to discover our body doesn't respond and perform at the same level each day. You soon learn what foods make it perform best, how sleep affects you and what role good hydration plays.

Years ago, I went on a weekend trip with a friend to the Great Smoky Mountains. We stayed in a motel and pledged to each other that we would keep our exercise routines intact even though we were traveling. In the early morning, we jumped into workout clothes and hit the parking lot of the motel, feeling a little conspicuous not having found a more appropriate place to exercise. Rounding the first lap, I looked up at the second story balcony. A man was standing there smoking and watching us work. He chose to sit on the sideline and wave. "Not working too hard up there," I thought to myself.

I no longer felt ridiculous exercising there, because I realized at that moment that *all of us are either participants or spectators in life's endeavors.* Choose to be a participant and you will have a new body and an abundant world in which to make that choice.

Target Heart Rate

Get out each day and try to get your heart rate elevated to an aerobic level for 20 to 40 minutes and building up to one hour. To find a safe range in which to exercise, establish your target heart rate. To do so, subtract your age from the number 220. The remainder is your "maximum heart rate." This is the maximum number of beats a minute your heart should reach while you are exercising, not more.

Multiply the remainder by .70 if you haven't exercised for a long time. If you exercise regularly, multiply the remainder by .75. This number is your "target heart rate". It represents the number of beats a minute you would like your heart to beat while you are exercising.

To determine your heart rate while exercising, place the tips of your index and middle fingers on your neck or on the inside of your wrist. Count your pulse for six seconds and multiply this number by 10. This is your heart rate while you have been doing your exercise.

Slow down if your heart rate exceeds the target rate you have set for yourself and, likewise, speed up a bit if your pulse drops below your target heart rate. Bringing your arms above your head as you walk increases your rate, as stated.

ACTION LIST:

➤ *Commit* yourself to a walking program. We all have busy lives. The way to keep your exercise promise is to make an appointment with yourself. Put it in on your calendar or in your PDA. Make it a part of your written agenda. Paste it on your refrigerator. If you were to make an appointment to meet a friend or a client at 6:00 PM you would be there. Just tell people you have an appointment. You do. It's with yourself.

➢ To lose weight, do 5-7 sessions a week. For weight maintenance, do 3-4 sessions a week.

➢ Stretch and slowly walk to warm up before you push yourself to your target heart rate.

➢ Pace yourself to build up to 15 minutes per mile.

➢ Cool down slowly after your walk.

➢ You no longer have to sit on the sideline watching. You are a participant!

[11]

Navigating Through
Food Landmines

"Our greatest glory is not in never falling, but in rising every time we fall."

– Confucius

At a support group meeting, a woman asked me, "How should I handle my eating at an upcoming wedding? I always seem to *pick* at foods until I have eaten many high calorie dishes!"

I put aside my intended topic and presented an elaborate list of skills and tips for handling eating in this circumstance. I also solicited suggestions from the rest of the group. The subject took most of the remaining time and the woman thanked us all profusely.

As I walked out of the meeting, she caught up with me. I asked her, "So, what skills did you learn and what are you going to do at the wedding about food?"

"Don't worry," she told me, "I'll just *pick*!"

Some of us have had so little control over our lives for so long that eating becomes the one arena where we can exert our control. Even though this woman asked for advice, she was not *committed* to amending her habits.

The people who do best with gastric bypass surgery follow the recommendations:

- Stick with the winners.

- Make best use of the Golden Period, so the weight comes off as quickly as possible and in good health.

- Follow the rules of the game: three meals, with protein first, then vegetable, then fruit.

- Take necessary vitamin supplements.

- Exercise.

- Drink water.

- Don't snack.

They have a huge emotional investment in all they have done for themselves, and deviation from their program is less appealing to them.

The Supermarket

Food shopping used to be a social event. People met their neighbors at the market and caught up on local news. For people with food issues, however, it is best to socialize elsewhere, and to keep the shopping session short.

Don't go unless you have to go and don't go there hungry. If you are hungry before you leave home, eat a few bites of scrambled egg.

Make a shopping list before you go and stick to it. You will spend less money on impulse items and you won't be tempted to buy unhealthy, empty-calorie snack foods.

Shopping with another bypass patient may help you both make healthy choices. Even better, ask your spouse if he would shop for you.

Go in, buy what is necessary and leave.

As you know, the inside structure of the market is rectangular in shape. The healthy foods you want ... fruits, vegetables, meats, yogurt, soy products, etc,... are all placed around the *perimeter.*

We are in the habit of "cruising" up and down the aisles believing that we somehow have to view all the goods once again. Let me assure you, the candy aisle is still there. So are all the other foods that we have eaten into obesity. *Don't cruise the aisles!*

Instead, shop the perimeter, then go down an aisle *if you must.* Pick up your item and return the same way.

For me, there is no bakery aisle in a market. I don't eat bakery products anymore, so why should I go down the aisle and be stimulated by the breads?

The thought that food is for others and not for me eventually triggers me to want to reward myself with food, usually within three days of feeling this deprivation. There must be a deprivation meter somewhere in my brain. *Without visual stimulation of the food, I don't feel deprived.*

By the way, have you ever noticed the contents of people's shopping carts when you are in line at the market? I have seen entire carts with nothing but processed foods in them. No fresh items at all, but just white bread, frozen dinners, candy, pastry and sugared cereals. How can anyone thrive on such food? Is it any wonder that so many Americans are malnourished and overweight?

"Deprived" Children?

Many times in support groups I hear people say they worry that their children will feel deprived if they can't have the foods in the house they are accustomed to eating. They fear their children will suffer if potato chips, cookies and candy are removed.

Here are some statistics on the generation of children our nation is raising:[15]

- In the 1970's, one in twenty children were obese. Now, one in three children are obese! 10% of children age 2 to 5 are obese.

- The average American child sees 10,000 food commercials each year, 95% of which are for fast foods, sugared cereals, candy and soft drinks.

"Childhood obesity and its co-morbidities present a very serious threat to the health, well-being and economics of future generations in this country and throughout the world. As many as one in three U.S. children may be overweight or obese and their 'fatness' increases the risk of diseases which, until recently, were considered extremely rare among children and adolescents. Such diseases include Type II diabetes, obstructive sleep apnea, gastritis and pancreatitis, fatty liver, increased cardiovascular risk factors and early signs of atherosclerosis (the vascular disease that causes heart attacks and strokes).[16]"

The cruelty children suffer due to the teasing of other children erodes their self-esteem like drops of boiling water dripping on a soft bar of soap.

Children respond to what parents teach and to the example they set. Convey a positive message about healthy eating. Allow children to make choices from among healthy foods in the house.

So, if your shopping cart has fresh meats, poultry and fish, different colored vegetables and some fruit, you can be proud that you have the self-esteem to feed your body well and to care lovingly for your family. Good for you!

Food Triggers

Are there certain *foods or smells* that always entice you? Food Triggers are signals that invite your eating even though you have no physical hunger. *Be aware of the fact that just the sight or association with these foods can begin an unwelcome episode of eating.*

Feelings can be triggers, too. When we are angry, we may want to eat crunchy junk food such as potato chips and pretzels. When we are sad, we may want to eat soft, comforting food, such as, ice cream and frozen yogurt.

You can count on these situations to be an antecedent to eating: *jealousy, boredom, loneliness, fatigue, anger and stress.*

Be aware of your triggers. For instance, if every time your mother calls, you end up feeling upset, which leads to an eating episode, acknowledge the cause and its effect. In this example, you now are aware that an unpleasant conversation with her precedes an eating episode. Therefore, be proactive rather than reactive. *You* choose the time for having the conversation. *You* place the call when you are feeling emotionally strong. Pick light-hearted topics to discuss, have a joke ready and avoid unpleasant topics that you know typically lead in a negative direction without a resolution. You have a lot in your power you can do to change attitudes and to affect behavior.

My friend Judy's mother, when asked how she was, always answered the question by asking, "So how could I be?"

Implied in the answer was that Judy wasn't doing enough to make her mother happy.

Don't ask the question in the first place if you know it will lead to frustration!

My friend, Joan, had a very difficult mother, who often argued and became obstinate when she didn't get her way. Joan then would eat to salve her hurt feelings. One day, after an argument at her mother's house, she devised a way to handle the situation differently from her normal pattern. Every day for a week, Joan would show up unannounced at her mother's house. She would ring the doorbell, hand her mother a rose and simply say, "I love you, Mom." Then she would turn away and go home. Nothing else. No discussion of the argument. No statement of who was right or wrong. Just a rose and an "I love you."

At the end of the week, Joan's mother greeted Joan with a hug and an invitation to come in. She told her daughter she couldn't even remember what the fight was about. She had been looking at her roses on the table all week and she had felt ashamed there was an argument at all. She cried as she told her daughter how much she loved her, too.

Joan took a "trigger" situation in hand and dealt with it directly. She didn't choose to eat food to cover up her frustration and pain. She understood how powerful love could be.

There are some people, however, who have no psychological mindedness, no insight and who place no value on peace. If you can affect no change in this triggering relationship, perhaps distancing yourself from that person is the best way to safeguard your program and your health.

Primary Foods

Primary foods are foods we learned to use early in our lives for *emotional comfort*. Mother gave us a cookie when we fell and skinned our knee. Or we were taken out for ice cream because someone at school hurt our feelings or we lost the ballgame. Solving problems by offering food as a reward, teaches children to seek sources outside themselves to salve emotional pain. It is good parenting to encourage them to discuss the event and to express their feelings, working towards a solution, rather than teaching children to stuff down their feelings with food. Expressing faith in your child's ability to solve problems enables her to feel masterful. She won't have to look for an external substance from the world in which to find solace.

Be sure you are not using primary foods as a bandage to cover up emotional pain. If you choose these comfort foods when you are in pain and have the belief that food will see you through, you reinforce the bond with the food and the bond grows stronger.

One of my primary foods is pizza. As a child, I would buy a pizza at the restaurant on the corner in times when I felt upset. Since I didn't want my parents to know what I had done, I would sit on the curb of a nearby street and eat the pizza with a friend.

I have too many primary associations with this food. I don't crave pizza now, but I will *never* allow it to come into my house. I don't even want to see an oil-stained pizza box in my refrigerator. I know better.

Ethnic Foods

Many ethnic foods are primary foods. I can still remember outings with my father to a Jewish bakery in our neighborhood. We would buy a huge, fresh, raisin-laden bran muffin and split it. His big, beefy hand would encircle my tiny one as we crossed the street and munched the muffin. It was our time together away from my sister and mother. We felt we had sneaked off to pull a caper. I loved him, and I loved our muffin outings that we shared together. I was the center of his attention. I felt his love and I felt safe. I will always identify that food with my father. It will always have an air of comfort for me and, therefore, be attractive even when I am not hungry.

There is no coincidence that I grew up to make great Jewish food. You know the kind. I invented recipes of such high fat content you could harness yourself to the back of a plow and till a 40-acre field to work off the calories! My cooking could clog an artery on the way down!

An Asian man cried to me one day, "There is no way can I live without white rice! My whole family eats it and I'm not going to be left out."

Rice is a primary food for him and he cannot imagine his life without it.

We discussed how powerful the rice has become in his thinking. He now eats his meals, *protein first, then vegetables* and less often, a little rice.

This man's rice, was my muffin, or maybe your spaghetti, or your baklava, or taco or other primary ethnic food.

Alcoholic Beverages

Not only are we unable to eat the same amount of food as we did before surgery, it is very unwise to drink alcoholic beverages as we previously had. Here are some reasons:

- I have been told by a surgeon that alcohol is the number one substance that post-operative patients use to cross-addict from food. That is, food addicts may substitute a different substance to mask the pain of emotional issues. Some others are drugs, sex, cigarettes, shopping, and relationships.

- I am hearing more and more about cirrhosis of the liver in post-operative patients. The majority of them had normal, although fatty livers before surgery. There is evidence that after weight loss surgery, alcohol appears to compromise the health of the livers of these people who drink too much.

- Alcohol burns as a sugar, inviting the release of insulin. You may dump.

- Alcohol is not the nutritious food you now need.

- Alcohol lowers your resistance to eating, adding extra calories.

- Alcohol peaks your appetite, especially for high fat foods.

- You will get drunk *much* faster since the alcohol enters your blood stream quicker than it did before your surgery. At one support group meeting, we were told of a police officer that had arrested several post-operative gastric bypass patients for drunkenness. Their blood alcohol level was over the legal limit. It is not the number of drinks or their size that is the problem, but rather how quickly the drink raises the blood level of alcohol.

Eating In Restaurants.

Now that you are getting back into a normal life, there are skills for maneuvering into your new world.

The Wave

Much of our socializing revolves around eating in restaurants. We use food for all our occasions, formal and casual.

For me, the fast food restaurant is a thing of the past. I need to eat the most nutritious food I can from now on.

When I go into a restaurant, my attitude is that I have rented the table for as long I am there. It is mine. Either I get my needs met or I leave. I am not encouraging rudeness. I am merely stating that if I can't assert even my food preferences, then how do I get my more sophisticated needs of life met?

Your server's objective is to maximize your bill, which increases the size of the tip you leave. So she begins to recite a list of the "specials" usually with highly descriptive prose. I immediately interrupt with a wave of my hand and say, "I am eating light." That's all. *A wave of my hand and a simple declaration* signals that I have made my decision and I don't need to be informed further. I teach it to support groups as *The Wave*. We all laugh, and they get the idea that they don't have to apologize for their choices nor ask approval for their needs.

When you do *The Wave*, there is no need to say that you are dieting or to tell your life history. There also is no need to state that you just had gastric bypass surgery and show a diagram of where all your digestive organs are now routed. Your life is none of your server's business and you don't have to apologize for yourself.

What about when your server asks about a dessert preference? I immediately interrupt with *The Wave* and say, "I am eating light." Try it yourself.

Divide and Conquer

When ordering, I ask at the same time that a take-home carton be provided at the time my meal is served. Let's say I want a steak. I order a great steak, despite the price (after all I'm going to eat it for two or more meals), double vegetables and, maybe, some fresh fruit for dessert.

When my meal comes, I divide the vegetables and steak in half, place one-half of the meal in the box and I put the box on the seat next to me. I am finished with the decision of how much of the meal to eat. If I were to allow the food to remain on my plate, I would be forced to deal with the temptation of eating the enormous portions served in American restaurants.

Normally at the table, you eat, fill up and stop. But, then the longer you sit there conversing with your friends, the more the remainder of your meal looks attractive. "Come and get me!" it calls.

As the food settles in your stomach and begins to be digested, there is more room for more food. You may start to pick at what's left on your plate. This episode of eating is no longer the same meal. *This eating is a snack!* In time, the day may come when you will be able to finish the entire meal at one sitting. Then, you may wonder why you had the surgery at all! Develop good habits now.

Note: I am not dieting when using the divide and conquer method. I choose to have the dinner I want. It always feels luxurious to me. I am satisfied. And, it is good value since I will have the remainder for another meal. When directed, your mind will follow your beliefs.

I end my meal by thanking the server for her consideration, and I leave a larger tip to encourage her to provide me the same service next time.

Become an observer of the restaurant habits of other people. Look at their food choices. Who is eating the double rack of ribs and the deep fat fried blooming onion? That person is not who you are any longer. You want a quality life, not to be "crawling after crumbs." You are strong and food cannot whip you around.

Salad Bars, Buffets and Parties.

Salad bars, buffets and parties are challenges because they provide tremendous visual stimulation to eat. Even if you are not hungry, the food somehow calls your name. I definitely avoid salad bars whenever possible.

If you go to a salad bar, buffet or a party, go with someone else. When you arrive, first look to see everything that is available. Then go to the front and pick up a plate. Tell your dining companion what you would like from the buffet and have your partner tell you his choices. Then proceed down the food aisle and select the appropriate portions and food... *for the other person.*

There is no way you would sabotage someone else's program by choosing the mayonnaise-laden pasta salad. And, your friend would not jeopardize your health by choosing the ice cream sundaes. Since we can only eat a small amount anyway, lusting after enormous mounds of food on the buffet table is ridiculous. Exchange plates, eat your meals *protein first, then vegetable then fruit,* and leave the scene of the buffet table.

It is surprising to me how good the first bite tastes, yet, how quickly the flavor wanes. Within the first five bites, my hunger is satisfied. Likewise, it surprises me how attractive the food looks when I am there and how quickly the vision fades from mind as soon as I leave the table. If you can put time, distance and a distraction between you and the food, you will find your mind will be elsewhere.

Never, ever eat to please someone else! Be polite, be firm and, if necessary, be gone.

When visiting someone else's house, there is nothing impolite about calling ahead to make sure there will be foods served that will be appropriate for you. If you had some other disease, wouldn't you ask those questions to preserve your health? You are just getting your needs met. I am not suggesting that people cook especially for you, just check to see there are some items on the menu from which you can choose and that you will enjoy. If not, explain you are there for their company and ask if you could bring some food for yourself. I have called caterers of weddings and hostesses of parties. If my questions are phrased tactfully, I find people are eager to help me. Sometimes I eat at home first and stay away from the buffet table at the party altogether.

While there, I walk around with a glass of water in my hand, so no one offers me a drink.

I once overheard a nurse advise a patient to accept a plate of food when it is offered at a party, carry it around until the hostess is out of sight and, then, abandon the plate. Food has an exaggerated appeal to us. If we carry food around, the temptation is to taste a little. Before long, most or all of the food is finished even if we didn't want it to begin with.

It is interesting to go to parties and observe people's relationship with food. At one party, I found all the women gathered around the buffet table discussing the many aspects of the food. It seemed they needed to touch it, discuss it, pat it and do everything but the Mexican Hat Dance on it. It was as if they could never be finished with the topic of food. After the party, they even wrapped portions for the guests to take home!

The men, on the other hand, had nothing to do with either the preparation, serving or clean up. They congregated in the den to discuss politics, sports and women. I joined them in the den and we had a great time. We laughed and teased each other about men's relationships with women.

Women are socialized to be the caretakers of the food, but the constant visual stimulation can lead to unwanted eating. Instead of residing at the food table, locate the most interesting person in the room to speak to.

Go up to a stranger at a party and say, "You look like an interesting person. I just wanted to talk to you for awhile." How could anyone resist being thought of as interesting? I did that at a party I attended in Peru. I met a man who was a physicist and who was interested in metaphysics. We spoke to each other the entire evening, exchanging stories and experiences. He really *was* interesting. Paul and I later attended a huge festival together in Cuzco. We joined a parade and danced like fools in the street! I saw Peru in a way I wouldn't have if I had not introduced myself to him and told him I thought he might be interesting.

Holidays

Many people find the holidays their greatest challenge. There are ways to avoid the food issue altogether.

One year, in order to bypass the usual Thanksgiving fare, my daughter and I bought tickets to see Shirley MacLaine perform. We had an extraordinary time. We didn't need the food to celebrate the holiday. After all, Shirley wasn't eating Thanksgiving dinner, either. We just had fun and we didn't feel deprived. We also didn't have huge quantities of Thanksgiving foods to deal with for the next week after the holiday.

Since most people have such high expectations of the perfect holiday that never transpires, changing the format and exploring other methods of celebration mean you might not be disappointed.

The holiday season will come and go. Most people gain 10 pounds over the holidays. I get excited knowing I will start the New Year thinner than I was the last year.

All the holiday fare will still be there if I choose, I tell myself. I am just on a *vacation* from these foods.

Traveling

When I get into the car, whether for a long trip, a business meeting, or even a drive to the market, I take along a package of soy cheese and some pea pods. Many times a short trip becomes extended and I can't tell you how many times I ate the soy cheese for my meal and avoided restaurants along the way.

Your self-esteem is everything! Protect your health program! It makes dealing with whatever other challenges life presents much easier.

ACTION LIST:

➤ Make a food landmine avoidance kit and designate a place for it in your car the way you would for a first aid kit. Include a plastic container large enough for half a restaurant meal, a bottle of water, bag of beef jerky and whatever else you need to protect yourself.

➤ Identify your primary foods and food triggers.

➤ Use *The Wave* at restaurants.

➤ Divide and conquer food portions each time you eat out.

Dispelling Old Beliefs

"All that we are is the result of what we have thought. The mind is everything. What we think, we become."

– Buddha

"Whether you think you can or whether you think you can't, you are absolutely right."

– Henry Ford

"I think I can. I think I can. I think I can."

– The Little Engine That Could

Your Surgeon Operated On Your Body, Not your Mind

The mind creates a plausible explanation of what we see. Whatever "holes" in the story that exist, the mind rushes in to complete the picture to make sense of it. It is often comical to watch this phenomenon take place.

One such example for myself was of a trip to the supermarket. I made my purchase and drove home. Upon unpacking the bags, I couldn't find an item. My mind quickly created a drama so the experience would make sense. I decided the checker was distracted and, therefore, hadn't placed the item in my bag. Mentally, I went through a trip back to the market, a discussion with the manager, a confrontation with the checker and much righteous indignation at my inconvenience. Then, I found the missing item in a bag that I had just folded. You see the story wasn't the truth, but only my mind's perception of the truth. We convince ourselves of any number of imaginary beliefs. Some reflect our values about food and about life in general.

At one weight loss surgery support group meeting, a woman had come to explore the possibility of having the surgery done. She turned to me and explained at length how sick she had been due to her obesity.

After hearing numerous success stories and accomplishments told by its proud members and their enthusiasm about the surgery, she then turned to me again and said, "If I can't have potatoes after I have this surgery, then I won't have it. I can't live without potatoes."

We are what we think.

Here are some "beliefs" people have told me:

"I *have* to taste something sweet at the end of my meal."

"If I am a guest at someone's house, I *have* to eat what is served or they will think I am rude."

"I *have* to have a snack at 10 PM. I've always done that."

"I *have* to eat often to keep up my strength."

"If it's in front of me, I *have* to eat it."

"I worked so hard today; I *have* to reward myself with food."

"I *have* to do everything perfectly."

"I *must* clean my plate or I'll be wasteful."

"I can't stand to ever be in pain and food makes me feel better."

"It's just another apple. Not too many calories. It's OK to have it as a snack. After all, I'm not eating cake."

"I *can't* go to the (movies/restaurant/travel) alone."

"Saturday night is date night. I *can't* go out without a date."

"I *can't* take care of myself alone."

"If I am thin, other people will expect too much from me."

"I am helpless. I just don't have any control."

"Men shouldn't cry."

"I can't afford to have what I want."

"Nice girls don't get angry."

"My needs don't matter."

"If I ignore that problem, it will go away."

The list is lengthy. You must have a few phrases you tell yourself that you are sure at the time must be true, as well. These beliefs perpetuate anxiety and create the need to soothe with food. They limit your life.

Be careful what you tell your mind. It thinks it is doctrine. Part of modifying your eating habits is to note the way you have structured language. Phrases like, "I have to," "I must," "I should" are very powerful, indeed. The mind wants to obey the declaration. The desperate statement of need sets up the feelings of deprivation and the result can be bingeing.

Bingeing

How much food is a binge? *It can be one bite of food eaten in a compulsive way.* You know when you are bingeing. There is no real physical hunger. You feel anxious. You make excuses to others so you can find a way to obtain what you want to eat. You create rituals that feel comfortable and familiar. Delaying your food gratification feels painful and anxiety-ridden. You have a strong sense of immediacy to have food.

In the planning and execution of the ritual binge, there is an arc of behavior that occurs. At the beginning of the arc, we feel anticipation and excitement over the upcoming eating event. At the top of the arc, there is relief while eating the food. As the arc continues downward, however, we feel shame, letdown and depression. So, what happens when we are depressed? We eat and the *binge cycle* repeats.

I remember all of the time and effort given to eating. Not just to the physical act, but to the planning of eating events. In my past, while engaged in conversation with someone, I appeared attentive to what he was saying when, in actuality, I was contemplating making a run to the nearest fast food restaurant. Food consumed me and I consumed it. It took up considerable hours in my day.

I created a world of isolation so I could be with my "substance." I created rituals around the planning, procuring and ingesting of food. I repeated those rituals in an habitual association with life events, so that, a trip home from the stress of work entailed a cruise through a fast food drive up. Even though my children were grown, I still ordered as if they were in the back seat. I performed the same rituals of opening the wrappers and preparing the food for eating. And, afterward, I defiantly tossed the wrappers in the same dumpster before I got home. The binge cycle then would repeat – anticipation, relief, shame and depression. Always and inevitably, there was depression.

Another example of food-preoccupation is the story of Amanda and her sister, Carol, both obese. They were too embarrassed to stand in line at the bakery, so they hatched a scheme: they called and ordered a sheet cake with, "Happy Birthday, Amanda" written on the top. Amanda and her sister then picked up the cake, parked around the corner, pulled out two forks and ate until they were close to vomiting.

In another story, a man I knew would order a 6-foot submarine sandwich and two large pizzas to be delivered to his home supposedly for a party. It was a party, all right. He ate alone, late into the night until he fell asleep in a stupor from food.

Many people have told me about throwing food into the trashcan in an effort to start a diet, only to retrieve it all later and eat it.

Does any of this behavior sound familiar to you?

I, myself, have hit several fast food restaurants in succession so I wouldn't be seen "shopping" for huge quantities of food at any one place, as if the whole world were paying attention to me anyway. I then brought home the multiple bags and devoured them alone. Food was my perfect companion. It gave me solace. It was my date on Saturday night. It made me feel defiant and powerful and in control of my own little world. Food became the accompaniment to my every event of living. The movies meant popcorn. An evening out meant dining in restaurants. In fact, I could hardly give someone street directions without a reference to food: "You go down this street and turn right at the ice cream store, keep going 'til you see the Mexican restaurant." You get the idea.

I know now that food was my companion, but *not* my friend.

Because you have had gastric bypass surgery, you have a new opportunity to break the binge cycle. You now have diminished appetite, early satiety, and greatly reduced obsessive thoughts and compulsivity towards food!

Without food problems to affect you directly or indirectly all day, there will be energy to spare for the exploration and enjoyment of other pursuits.

The Old Rules No Longer Apply

The rules we learned in our childhood to protect ourselves from a threat often work against the behavior we need to do to recover our health.

"Our *mistaken* survival tactics include:

- Always putting others first.

- Fixing problems for everybody else in the hope that they'll reach back to us.

- Keeping everyone happy.

- Not feeling or showing anger or sadness. Or both.

- Looking put-together.

- Being very responsible.

- Not making mistakes.

- Not troubling others.

- Being brave.

- Being invisible.

- Keeping our feelings under control at all times.

Whenever we break a survival rule we feel scared and anxious, so scared and anxious that we eat. The paradox is that to recover, we need to break these rules. Breaking these rules creates such discomfort, however, that we want to cling to the only consistent comfort we know—food.

It takes time to learn to break these rules. We must be kind to ourselves. The penalty for unkindness to ourselves is almost always a drive to eat. Whether we like the idea or not, to recover, we must learn self-kindness. That's different from self-indulgence."[3]

Do any of these methods of looking at life appear familiar to you?

Recognize how much you shy away from activities and people just because the situation feels uncomfortable. Let yourself linger in a little discomfort so you can witness your own ability to cope and to triumph.

As the weight started coming off, I made a conscious effort to force myself to deal with uncomfortable situations instead of avoiding them. The most difficult situations for me were social gatherings. I wanted to stay home, safe and sound. I wanted to be comfortable. But I didn't learn much about myself by staying home. I needed interaction with other people to learn both about myself and about the world.

Let's say you are invited to a party where you only know the hostess. You fear she will be busy with her guests and you might have to fend for yourself among strangers. In the past, when the invitation was extended, you might have avoided going by saying, "I'll try to make it."

"I'll try" is just a way of saying, "I don't want to face telling you this on the phone, but I'm not going to show up." It is like "trying" to pick up a piece of paper. You either pick it up or you don't.

Instead, go to the party and accept that you might be uncomfortable at first. Most of us are. Remember, you can be any "you" that you want to be. You can sit and observe people, or you can mingle and chat. See how long it takes before you feel comfortable. I bet it happens in less time than you think it will.

At a party, I look for someone who is uneasy as well. I strike up a conversation with that person. Soon we are both at ease and I have made a friend.

I attended a conference where a psychiatrist told a story about a cocktail party invitation he accepted. He sat on the couch chatting for an entire evening with a man whose acquaintance he had just made. The two of them had many interests in common and they enjoyed each other's company. At the end of the evening the man asked the psychiatrist, "By the way, what do you do for a living"?

When the man learned, he exclaimed, "Oh, if I had known you were a psychiatrist, I would never have sat down next to you!"

Just get to know people.

No More Isolation

As I became more and more obese, I endured the burden day by day until the pain became unbearable. Consequently, I entered into an intimate dance with food, isolating myself more and more away from the world. The result was unimaginable loneliness.

Now, I welcome people into my life. I find joy in relating to others. I wonder what their lives might be like. Often I'll ask them. Even peripheral relationships are important to me. In exchanging pleasantries with different shop owners, for instance, I feel connected. I feel recognized in my own community and a part of life.

I measure time differently now. I look at my loved ones and tell them how much they mean to me. I savor tiny changes in nature. I laugh more. I appreciate more. I am prepared for more.

It is vital to your recovery that you replace the relationship you have created with food with a relationship with people.

The Old Behaviors

"Insanity is repeating the same behavior and expecting a different result."

– Paul Ehrlich

It takes brutal honesty to look at old behavioral patterns and to weed out the ones that lead to weight gain. For instance, we know that obesity is a progressive disease. What seems like a harmless "bit of this" eaten on one occasion, leads to repetition of the eating until a habit is created, consuming larger amounts.

Remember the jingle? "Betcha can't eat just one!"

Here's how food-to-event associations work. Let's say I get home from work at 5:00 PM each day. I want to relax from the day's stress, so I turn on the TV. A food commercial flashes on the screen. I automatically get up and go to the refrigerator. There are salad and cake inside. I decide to "be good" and eat the salad instead of the cake. How many days do you think I might repeat that behavior before I decided I deserved the cake?

The stimulus was the need to reward myself for a day's work and the commercial showed me how. The reaction was to go to the refrigerator for my reward, rather than finding other pursuits. If you answer that stimulation-reward routine each time, the association of the event with food grows stronger. Each time, that cake looms more and more inviting. The habit will be set in place and soon the salad will be replaced with cake. In other words, it is not the *type* of food chosen to snack on, but rather it is the strong bond created with the stimulation to eat in that time and circumstance and the consumption of the food.

If you doubt this statement, imagine going out to the movies. Does the idea of buying popcorn and candy accompany that thought? Some other associations of an event with eating include going to a ballgame and eating a hot dog, watching TV while eating a sandwich, attending a Super Bowl party and consuming beer and snacks, and so on, all making an association of the event with an episode of eating.

Although it is uncomfortable in the beginning, go to an event to enjoy it for its own sake, not to have justification to eat. When you go to a party, for instance, notice who is in the middle of the room laughing and talking with others? Isn't it usually the people who are not so invested in food that they can bear to leave the buffet table? They are enjoying themselves without the constant consumption of food. Force yourself to do the same and soon the food association weakens.

Emotions

Much of the eating we do as obese people is born out of the desire to soothe our emotions.

David Viscott wrote[17]

"*Hurt* is what we feel when we experience a loss.

Anxiety is what we feel when we anticipate a loss.

Anger is what we feel when we resent a loss.

Depression is what we feel when we are depleted by our loss.

Guilt is what we feel when we internalize our anger and feel worthless because of the loss."

We experience loss many times a day. We experience loss when we feel embarrassed or when someone criticizes us, not just the usual association of loss of someone through death. Many times, when we feel a sense of loss, we associate the event with the need to soothe with food. There is not any connection to physical hunger. It is in seeing how we have attached food to events and to the feelings of loss that we understand the misuse of food and the resultant obesity.

"To be proactive instead of reactive is to recognize your feelings in response to the stressor, but also to think and choose the most effective behavior needed to take care of the stressor. If a stressor triggers anger, you carefully choose behavior that will respond to the stressor and end your anger. If a stressor triggers hurt, you carefully choose behavior that will respond to the stressor and end your hurt. If a stressor triggers fear, you carefully choose behavior that will respond to the stressor and end your fear. Behavior that is based on thought and careful choice resolves the stressor and leaves us feeling emotionally free."[18]

Remember the story of Joan and her mother? She learned to deal directly with the emotion and not to eat over it. That's real power.

Being Truly Alive

There is a saying I love:

"If someone or something does not bring you alive, it is too small for you." (author unknown)

Look to be brought alive by the world and to bring your world alive. Notice that when you feel expansive, smiling, enriched, sustained, energetic, of a generous heart and stimulated, you are brought alive.

If you are closed down emotionally, smaller in generosity than you would like to be, diminished, fearful, sad, making excuses, hurt and/or sabotaged and betrayed, most likely those messages from your body are telling you that the situation and/or person affecting these feelings is too small and not right for you.

Life Purpose

All my life, I have been terrified of public speaking. The thought of an audience looking at me, especially at my body without a podium to hide me, was so frightening I could feel adrenaline coursing through my veins. I would perspire, my voice would shake and I couldn't calm down to deliver my speech.

One of my constant prayers has been to be able to find my purpose in life and to express it well to the world. At this time, I am conducting gastric bypass surgery support groups, educating patients about how to adapt before and after their surgery and sharing this knowledge and experience with you. I am planning seminars. When I speak in front of people, I feel I can embrace them and be embraced by them. I share my personal stories and I feel no embarrassment to disclose my exodus from obesity, full of triumphs and of failures. This is who I was. This is who I am.

Our anger at the world grows when we are ignorant of our life's purpose and the inability to realize our goals. We have been excluded both by others and by our own limitations from reaching to find out who we are and what we must do.

I think of the artisan who spends months creating a beautiful musical instrument, a painter expressing an image, an opera singer caught in the rapture of her music, all in their passion and I know they are "in love."

This exodus from obesity allows a body that will carry the spirit where it wants to go. We have the opportunity to rid ourselves of the anger associated with a restricted life. We can examine our own possibilities. We then can express these talents to make ourselves happy and the side effect is the enrichment of others.

As the weight melts away examine what your life is about and how you want it to express your passion and life purpose. Is it possible to be caught in one's rapture and to feel unsatisfied and angry at the same time? I don't think so.

I have learned not to be in awe of others. Each of us possesses gifts in life. But each person also has parts of herself she hasn't developed. Maybe a person is a great pianist, but a lousy husband. Maybe she can sell real estate, but she has no skills for creating a warm and loving home of her own. He is a math whiz, but can he bake a cherry pie? Get it? Each person has both developed and undeveloped aspects of personality and every house on the block its problems, even if we can't see them. No one lives a completely charmed life without challenges.

A Goddess Party

I once read a quote by Pablo Picasso, "There are only two kinds of women– goddesses and doormats."

I hated that quote when I first encountered it. It made me struggle inside. But, I thought about it long and hard.

I finally decided to host a Goddess Party. I bought Miss Piggy cups and napkins and balloons. Each person I invited showed up as the goddess of her choice. The costumes were wild and imaginative. We extolled how wonderful it was to be female and that if Picasso thought there were only two types of women, we certainly knew which one we were going to be!

ACTION LIST:

➤ Make a list of myths you tell yourself. Challenge their legitimacy in your life now. Which ones are impeding your development?

➤ Define your life purpose. What would it be? How can you achieve this goal?

➤ Anyone up for a Goddess Party?

[13]

Dealing With Fat Prejudice

"The sectarian thinks he has the sea ladled into his private pond."

Tagore (Fireflies)

"Our culture is steeped in messages that thin is in, despise size. We've come to accept the idea of abusing ourselves with self-hate and crazy diets. We avoid desired activities as if we agree that we are members of an inferior society."[3]

In exploring the subject of fat prejudice, let's first examine how *we* have been conditioned to regard obesity, that is, how we consider others and ourselves. Here are questions to ponder: Do you have your own biases against obese people? Do you discriminate against them and hold preconceived, negative judgments about them? Are you emotionally invested in keeping someone else "fat"? Do you look for the negative qualities in others?

In facing the possibility of our own biases, we can begin to see how others have developed theirs. Understanding how prejudice is born and nurtured puts us on a road to forgiveness.

It was difficult for me, at first, to forgive people's insensitivity toward me as an obese person. I felt injured and misunderstood.

As an example, I remember lying in the hospital prepared to face my gastric bypass surgery and ready to be wheeled into the operating room. A man approached my bed, pulled down my sheet, looked at my legs and stated, "You have very heavy thighs. They are the kind of thighs that will take a lot of work." He turned away and left. I don't know to this day, who he was or why he thought he had the right to invade my privacy and speak to me that way.

Now I understand that we are all conditioned in life to fear what is unfamiliar and to form impressions, negative as they might be, without justification. We listen to and perpetuate stereotype. We all have prejudices that we must challenge.

In forgiving that man's trespass, I can expend my energy in more positive directions.

Obesity Is Determined Genetically

Before we are persuaded to think that obesity is a character disorder, it is helpful to know that it is genetically determined the way hair, skin or eye color is. Yet, fat prejudice pervades our society. We are robbed of our self-respect for the misfortune of having a genetic disease. Obese people frequently encounter social abuse and often are taken less seriously by the medical community when it comes to treatment.

As obese individuals, we felt this prejudice intensely and to the core of our being. We wished that people see us for who we really were inside instead of what we looked like on the outside. Now, with the weight off, we feel *angry* that the same people that avoided us and found us less worthy when we were obese are friendly and accepting of us now. A part of our new lifestyle change is dealing with the fat prejudice of others.

In our exodus from obesity, we may pass though some very angry feelings towards the world and its insistence that because of our size we were somehow less worthy. The anger is understandable. We want to rail against the pain we have felt for so long when we looked into someone's eyes and realized they saw us in a diminished way. When we are a normal weight, we may wish to retaliate.

Society has been inculcated to see the obese in very negative terms. But *we* feel we are exactly the same fat or thin. As we lose the weight, however, we learn to deal with fat prejudice by recognizing that we are *not exactly* the same people now as we were when we were obese. Weight loss brings us added energy, more positive thought, the agility to be a partner in activities and a greater availability to others. Before, we structured our lives around sedentary activities. We are more physically active now. We are more emotionally open. Other people notice that and they are attracted to our energy, to our elevated mood and outlook. People are reacting to who we are now.

"You are not the same person! You are not the same person! You have changed your eating habits, which has affected your schedule, your finances, your wardrobe and your interest in your personal appearance. And the dominoes continue to fall. You smile more, you exude greater confidence, you don't mind being noticed as much, you react a little more boldly than before and you are able to do many things you never considered when you were large. So, you are *not* the same individual! Overweight, you felt awkward and embarrassed, got angry when victimized on an airplane or at a restaurant. Overweight, you couldn't ride in a roller coaster or run a marathon.

The thin you is an evolution of the fat you. Not a reproduction. Do not be misguided by well meaning phrases from your old way of thinking.

Anger is the number one issue that comes up in my sessions with clients exploring the long-term weight loss phenomena. We experience anger at others for discriminating against us because we are fat.

Your anger will reveal itself on your body. Anger is a powerful emotion that cannot be hidden for long periods of time. Sooner or later, your anger will eat at you until you have gained back every pound you thought you lost. Let it go. Find purpose and find peace, but do not replace food with anger. It will destroy you.

My self-esteem has become so important to me that I have to let go from my life anyone who makes me struggle in the belief of myself." [19]

Maybe we can learn to forgive the insensitivity of those who have been conditioned in their prejudice of the obese. Maybe we could educate people and sensitize them to the suffering this disease causes. In other words, let's become role models so that "fat jokes" and other cruel comments are never allowed in our presence. Open a door for whomever is behind you. Offer obese people your smile. Look at obese people directly, not past them, as it is painful to be regarded as invisible. Seek the potential and purpose in obese people. Forgive, because it will release you of negative energy that can be placed positively elsewhere. Make obese people feel welcome in your presence as you would in your home.

ACTION LIST

➢ Find three ways to remedy fat prejudice in your home, job or community.

[14]

Restructuring Relationships

"Between the shores of Me and Thee there is the loud ocean, my own surging self, which I long to cross."

Tagore (Fireflies)

At one time in my life, I had a friend, Rosalyn. We often ate lunches out together. As we dined, we shared our heart's problems and the trials and tribulations of our day. When I announced I was going to Durham, North Carolina to a lifestyle and weight loss program, she flew into a rage and yelled, "You are so selfish! All you think about is yourself!"

Threatened by the possibility I might become more attractive, she destroyed the relationship. That was the last time I saw her.

Restructuring Relationships With Others

When you lose weight, you change before people's eyes in many ways and this can be unsettling to them. As you regain your self-esteem, you are more assertive of your needs and stronger in the world. This change can threaten a relationship that is based on your compliance and subservience.

In one of my support group sessions, I remember hearing of an average weight man that was married to a woman weighing 400 pounds. He constantly berated her for her size, demeaning her in her failed attempts to lose weight. Finally, she decided to please him and to change her life. In despair, she had gastric bypass surgery and lost most of her excess weight. Her husband then divorced her. When he remarried, he chose another 400-pound woman!

Carla and Ron had their own marital dance. They were on "diets together." Carla, trying with all her might to lose weight, was making strides far beyond her husband's attempts at weight loss. He felt left behind. One night, at midnight, Ron crept into their bedroom with a tray full of lasagna. He waved it under Carla's nose and awakened her with the aroma. He then pulled out two forks. Carla ate with Ron and abandoned all her efforts at weight loss after that. Having obesity in common somehow had stabilized their marriage.

These stories illustrate why you need to restructure your relationships as you lose weight.

Consider your friends, loved ones and your co-workers at this time. If you have not yet had the gastric bypass surgery, all the people in your life are in a relationship with an obese person ... *you.*

After surgery, you may find that some people were more comfortable with the obese you. To your married friend, you may now be a sexual threat because she feels her husband is attracted to you. To your co-workers, you may now be a serious contender for the next job promotion. Your husband, who always avowed to love you "fat", now worries about your attractiveness to other men and fears you may abandon him.

Generally, after weight loss surgery, it is found that good marriages are enhanced by the weight loss and that unhealthy ones drift apart.

You know before anyone else that you are changing and you have had more time to adjust to the change than others have had. Sometimes, all people need is a chance to catch up. It is like finding out you are pregnant and keeping it a secret for a few months. You have had time to adjust to your new self. Then you reveal your secret, your changing body and attitudes and the world hasn't yet known you are different. Give people the benefit of the doubt that they do have your best interest at heart. Give them some time to come around. Assure them whether you are obese or normal weight you still love them. Tell them how they can assist you in your weight loss efforts. Give them the opportunity to be their best selves.

However, if in the end someone can't support, appreciate and accept you at a normal, healthy weight, perhaps that person is better out of your life.

Restructuring Relationship With Yourself

There is a passage in the Bible:

> "Do not hide your light under a bushel basket. Let people see your good works so they can give praise to your Father in heaven" (Matthew 5:14-16). "

Our light is to be placed as a "beacon on a hill." Let others see your light.

Another quote:

> "Our deepest fear is not that we are inadequate. Our deepest fear is that we are powerful beyond measure. It is our light, not our darkness, that most frightens us. We ask ourselves, who am I to be brilliant, gorgeous, talented and fabulous? Actually who are you not to be? You are a child of God. Your playing small doesn't serve the world. There is nothing enlightened about shrinking so that other people won't feel insecure around you. And as we

let our own light shine, we unconsciously give others permission to do the same. As we are liberated from our own fear, our presence automatically liberates others."

– Nelson Mandela (inaugural speech, 1994,
Written by Marianne Williamson)

I have met hundreds of people of size. I find, generally, that many have compensated in other areas of their lives for their perceived lack of personal attractiveness. Many are highly educated or accomplished in diverse areas. I have heard these obese people cry that they have mastered so much of their lives and, yet, here they are with a "weight problem" that hangs over their heads and shadows their lives.

I am learning more and more everyday that I have been guided to concentrate on my strengths. And I will not be less than I am for anyone. Hopefully, neither will you.

We have faced the fear of surgery. We have dealt with weight loss. We have uncovered the core issues and problems that were hiding under the surface of our eating. It is time to recognize and to emphasize the strengths of our personalities, to appreciate our selves and to shine. Restructuring of our conceptual image is part of the work as well as the physical image.

"In the depth of winter, I finally learned that within me lay an invincible summer."

– Albert Camus

Within you lies an invincible summer, too.

ACTION LIST:

➤ Say out loud and complete the following sentences:

- "I am very good at ...."

- "I shine and come alive when I ...."

- "I feel powerful when I................."

➤ You have lost weight and are out in the world. You are dealing with people of all shapes and sizes. This is a good time for a second *Dear Me Letter*. Who am I now? How have I changed in relation to myself before surgery? You are creating a new you in more ways than one. A new *Dear Me Letter* would give you a basis for comparison. How would you answer these questions:

- Describe how you have changed.

- What are your dreams and how are you achieving them?

- What is it like to live in your new body?

- What are you learning, discovering, exploring?

- Who are the people around you?

- How do you define health for yourself?

- What are you looking forward to?

- How are you conquering your fears?

- What interests that you had wished for when you were obese are you pursuing now?

- Are you becoming brave?

- Can you allow yourself to be placed in uncomfortable positions so you can grow?

- Do you still stay home alone or are you getting out and learning about yourself in relation to the world?

- Are you finding your life's purpose?

[15]

Adapting to Your New Image

"Mirror, mirror on the wall – "

– The witch in "Sleeping Beauty"

This Space Is Unoccupied

When you lose weight rapidly, the changing size, contour and perception of your body can be disorienting.

Over the years, we learned the amount of room we needed to occupy and made provisions to accommodate our size. We have ingrained in our minds an image of what we look like that includes how we fit on furniture and through doors. Now we are surprised when we catch a glimpse of our reflected selves. We now face an ever-changing form.

A weight loss surgery friend and I used to engage in an activity we called our "mall therapy." Seated in a shopping mall, we would ask each other how we saw the other in relation to a passerby.

"Am I larger or smaller than she is?"

"Is my (whatever body part) larger or smaller than hers?"

This activity was not done to be unkind. We actually didn't know how we looked in relation to others and needed someone else's perspective. It helped us to understand where we fit in and how far we had to go. In other words, our weight scale didn't give us enough information to provide a consistent image in our brain. We needed a visual indicator, a frame of reference. Eventually, we got to the point where we could rely on our ability to see ourselves realistically.

Soft cushions on our body are giving way to bony prominences. Large, rather undefined areas are taking form. Clothes hang differently. We feel more exposed ... and we are. We have trouble seeing ourselves in relation to other people and where in the diverse graduation of human sizes we fit.

Our brain cannot adapt quickly to the rapid change. A psychologist explained to me it that takes two to three years to grasp a dependable understanding of one's new image.

For slender people, their so-called "fat day" means they ate too much last night and they feel bloated in the morning. For us, we may imagine that overnight we have gained all our weight back. Disoriented in our lack of a reliable sense of perception and information about ourselves, this discomfort is part of the normal course and will eventually find resolution. Here are some reliable markers:

- People will regard you differently. There will be comments and opinions. The way people look at us has become part of our own self-image.

- The mirror, obviously, reflects the changes, but our mood will interpret how we see that image through a filtered impression. More than once I have heard people say, "I'm having a fat and ugly day."

- You will get a new tactile understanding of your body. I remember waking up one morning and running my hand over my side. I felt a bump and feared I had a tumor. What a nice surprise to learn I had a hipbone!

In Surgery For the Morbidly Obese Patient, Dr. Deitel writes, "All the senses contribute to the perceptual aspect of body image but the tactile and kinesthetic senses seem to be the most important."

- Your clothes will give you feedback. It is time to stop wearing garments that stretch to the next county! The use of expanding waistbands allows the image confusion to continue. I find that jeans are unforgiving. If my jeans are tight, my weight is up.

- We come to see ourselves as more sexually defined and appealing. For some of us, that will be a welcomed benefit. For others, it will send them running for the hills, sabotaging their weight loss efforts out of fear of having to confront their sexual attractiveness.

- The scale, tape measure and weight graph provide testimonies.

As our size diminishes, we may feel that we are "wasting away." We wonder if we are becoming less powerful, smaller and more insignificant in the world. Some people feel strong only if they can physically command more space.

Twenty years ago, I made a great friend, Tessie. Tiny of stature, she might have weighed 100 pounds on a good day. Tessie is the best doctor I have ever had the privilege of working with. She was "born" to be a physician and healer, and my respect for her is profound. Her stature doesn't stop her. She obtains the results she needs with calm self-assurance, clear and concise direction and good leadership. She doesn't take up much space, but she can certainly command hers. My point is that we do not have to be large to be taken seriously.

Visual Testimony

Taking periodic pictures as you are losing weight, not just the two "before and after" ones, gives you a better sense of your changing size. When you place those pictures, side-by-side, your mind more easily conceptualizes your rapid change.

Image Distortion

In observing the American vision of so-called physical beauty and health, I see a perversion of body image and a depiction that I feel is unrealistic and unhealthy.

One school study showed silhouetted images of female and male forms that were graduated from underweight to grossly overweight to groups of women and men separately. It asked them to select the preferred shapes.

The results showed that women had an acceptable image norm for themselves that was very much thinner than what men had for women. That is, women liked the thinner silhouette of women and men liked a heavier one. The conclusion is that most men do not want women pencil-thin, but women think they do, and we have perpetuated the myth that "you can never be too thin."

Men, on the other hand, chose the heavier silhouette as acceptable for themselves and women agreed with that choice. The conclusion is that men are valued more in our society for attributes other than their thinness.

Children exhibit a prejudice against obesity as early as age four. Our society is obsessed with the thin body. Magazine ads extol the thin female form. Many of the models in magazines are in their mid-teens. Are they a realistic standard for us? Images of the models are altered for the camera. Cindy Crawford courageously stated on TV one night, "Even *I* don't look like Cindy Crawford!"

Set Realistic Goal Weights and Expectations

Because we no longer have a strong sense of our body, we may set a goal weight that is completely unrealistic and unhealthy for ourselves.

The first time I began a significant weight loss program, I decided ahead of time that I should attain my college weight. I might just as well have tried to attain my birth weight! I had entered college at the age of 17, when I weighed less than 120 pounds. My bones hadn't even stopped growing then! If I weighed that now, at my height and age, I would look gaunt and ill. My collarbones would probably collect rainwater!

I like having a body that looks a little rounded and womanly. I also know what weight is comfortable for me to maintain, which allows me to enjoy food and not to have to be "dieting". My current BMI is in the normal range. I try to dress with simplicity and elegance. I have no illusions that I am not the ingénue that entered college so many years ago, and it would deny the woman I have become now with my years of wisdom and experience to try to be her.

How long has it been since you have been all the way down in weight? Do you have an image that is much too thin or much too young? Women and men, alike, want to remember their college days and "relive them thin" by aiming for a physical goal that is unhealthy and unsuited to age.

Pick a target *range* of weight according to the normal BMI range for your height. And, when people ask you what your goal weight is, you tell them you will know when you get there!

Where's My Report Card?

Initially, compliments come swiftly and often. There will come a day, however, when people have made their adjustment to our new image and they stop commenting on it. It is at this time, when we feel we have lost the limelight. Life is just the usual "day-to-day." We feel vulnerable and we may sabotage our own efforts. It is imperative that we learn what pleases us, to work for our own approval. We note our own milestones and accomplishments and give ourselves a "report card"!

Life recedes to the ordinary activities that normal weighted people encounter in their lives, since they are not having a major life event happen to them as you have been experiencing. They already know what you are learning – that being normal weight does not preclude life's problems and the learning of life's lessons. It just takes a major obstacle out of the way.

The Benefits of Being Fat

I have heard the statement, "Sometimes I miss being fat," from patients.

Carl Jung stated, *"All situations have both plusses and minuses."*

What, then, are the "plusses" of being fat?

- Less is expected of me.

- I can count on food to be there for me, whereas people are unpredictable.

- Being fat means I know the territory and I feel safe.

- I don't have to deal with my own attractiveness to others.

- I don't have to change my habits.

It is not unusual to feel this way from time to time during your weight loss.

I generally find, however, that people are greatly pleased with the results of their surgery and they are darn glad they had it.

Self Concept—Your Essence

I want to challenge you with an exercise. It was given to me years ago and, I must say, it was one of the most difficult assignments I have ever had to write. Limited to one paragraph, write your essence, everything that is your most innate you. These characteristics are your "bare bones," so to speak, the core of you that must be in place for you to feel in your personality.

From this exercise you will learn to identify your core self. You will also realize that if you have met someone who demands you to be less than this "essence," you will not be able to be with that individual. This core of yourself is who you are and must be.

Not to influence your own answer, but I will tell you that a part of my essence is to be kind. It is important to me. I try to give people the right of way on the road, the benefit of the doubt, an ear to their problem, etc. That is how I put myself into the world.

See? From my understanding of my essence comes a way to structure my behavior.

ACTION LIST

➢ Create a "Positive Image" page in your journal.

➢ Keep track of your time in the limelight, people's comments and reactions to you, etc.

➢ Set some goals for your growth that will give you a sense of mastery in accomplishment.

➢ In one paragraph, and in only one, write your essence. This essence that you describe must contain essential characteristics without which you would not be "you".

200 Pleasurable Things
To Do Instead Of Eating

"A dream is a wish your heart makes...."

Cinderella,
Lyrics: Mack David, Al Hoffman.

When I introduce the topic *200 Pleasurable Things To Do Instead Of Eating* in my weight loss surgery support groups, I wear an oversized, multi-colored, court jester's hat, with balls hanging from it. As we go around the room, each person volunteers to wear the hat and to read one alphabetical section from the list. Then I ask if there are any more ideas we can think of for enjoyable things to do that start with the letter we are on. The hat is passed and we laugh at how funny we look in it. It feels good for us to be laughing at ourselves for a change and also to see there is more to life than eating.

However, there are two serious reasons why I introduce this activity:

- *In order to lose weight and to keep it off, it is necessary to have a collection of pleasurable activities to replace the recreational eating that you used to engage in.* These activities, your interests and other rewards will allow you to broaden your horizons, have fun and become a more interesting and accomplished person. Not coincidentally, you also will be a long way from your refrigerator.

- *The crux of recovery from food addiction, or any addiction, is to change our allies.* We must learn to turn away from food and towards relationships with people. *Ritual eating* is usually done in private. I don't think I ever invited someone to my home saying, "Come on over, I'm planning to binge and eat everything in sight!" My *only partner* was food. It is crucial to diminish the allure and power of food and to accentuate an outward exchange with other people. And it is crucial to be fulfilling your life purpose since many times food is the substitute for unfulfilled aspirations.

So here with some whimsy, yet with serious encouragement, is my list of 200, or so, pleasurable things to do instead of eating:

A—acting, archery, art, astronomy, astrology, African dance, aquariums, antiquing, aerobics, animal rights, (patient) advocate, auctions, acrobatics, art collecting, arm wrestling, aroma therapy, archeology, Angel (for your support group).

B—ballooning, boating, backgammon, baseball, basketball, basket-weaving, badminton, baton-twirling, bird-watching, belly-dancing, ballet, body-surfing, break-dancing, bowling, beach-walking, be a big brother, board game, book, balance checkbook, brush your teeth.

C—cartwheels, canoeing, camping, crafts, courting, clogging, (garage)cleaning, comedy, croquet, create a bird sanctuary, collecting, crewel stitchery, cross-country ski, cards, crochet, catamaran, concert, (buy a) CD.

D—darts, day-trips, dream, dog training, decorate, design clothes, furniture, etc., date, dune buggy, dance wherever you hear music, (watch the) dawn, donate to charity.

E—earth science, Egyptology, egg decorating, exercise.

F– fundraising, fortune-telling, flower arranging, furniture refinishing, football, folk dancing, folk music, fishing, flirting, flying, (be a) friend, fair, festival, fix something, frame pictures.

G—garden, grow herbs, guitar, (become the) gift you give to someone else, garage sales, get glamorous, (buy a) gift.

H—horseback riding, hiking, homeowners association, host a street dance, hang gliding, harmonica playing, horse around with your dog, kids, hobby.

I—Imax theatre, investing club, invent something, introduce people, inspire people, imagery.

J—jump rope, jog, jazz dancing, jewelry making, journal.

K—kayaking, kite flying, knitting, kissing, kitten.

L—library, learn an instrument, learn a language, learn the names of flowers and trees, love someone well, leap for joy, listen well, laundry.

M—mountain trips, magic, movies, martial arts, meet neighbor, make someone laugh, museums, massage, music, make love, mystery trip.

N—nature walks, nap, naturalist talks, name state capitals, needlepoint.

O—observe people, orchestrate a car rally, (play an) oboe.

P—pray, piano, politics, parasail, paint projects, go to a play, photography, ping-pong, public speaking, plant a tree for the next generation, (day at the) park, puppy, pedometer, (buy) plants, palm reading, plan a party.

Q—quiet reflection, quilting.

R—racquetball, railroads, reading, racing, rake the yard, read both sides of an argument, rock-climbing, rock and roll, reggae, romantic walk.

S—sculpt, sew, swim, stagecraft, story-telling, study, star gaze, snow board, shell-collecting, square dancing, sailing, step-dancing, squash, shoe shopping, ski, skate, skip, self-defense course, surfing, snorkeling, send some flowers, sport, singing, surprise party, see the sunset, scrapbooks.

T—tap dance, trampoline, travel, tennis, tango, teach remedial reading, thrift store shopping, thank you cards, treadmill club.

U—ukulele.

V—volunteer, voice lessons, vacation, visit your neighbor.

W—western dancing, weight lifting, walking (power), long distance, wash and wax your car, wallpaper, wood working, work at something you love, whale-watching, white water rafting, (create a) walking club, weaving, window shop, water aerobics.

X—help?

Y—yard sales, yodeling, yard work, yoga.

Z—zoo, zoology.

Can you see life opening up for you? In this world of abundance, there are treasures awaiting you. With courage, imagination and now a body that will take you to new places, you can soar.

ACTION LIST

➤ Make a personalized list of the pleasurable things *you* will do instead of eating.

➤ Start doing them.

[17]

Celebrating Your New Life

"Make your life come true."

– Gregg Lavoy

"Work like you don't need money.
Love like you've never been hurt.
Dance like no one's watching"

– Satchmo Paige

Learning Celebration

In the Jewish religion, it is the tradition to bury the deceased within 24 hours of death. The only event I know of that overrides and delays a burial is a wedding. Jews are charged by God to celebrate life first and foremost. There is so much in life to celebrate and to enjoy.

In this spirit of celebration, I especially love to visit my daughter who lives in Paris with her husband. The French culture celebrates life. Any circumstance it seems is a cause for celebration. If you have ever been exposed to French hospitality, you will know what gracious hosting is all about.

When I visit, my daughter's mother-in-law, Maguy, creates a meal that is gracious, beautiful and delicious. I always feel honored to be seated at her table. More importantly, Maguy shares with me something in her life, her porcelain collection, for example, or her books on gardens, antiquities, her artwork, anything that gives me a glimpse into her enjoyment of life.

My daughter's father-in-law, Manu, is a magnificent host. He, at one such a dinner, opened a delicious bottle of wine. Before I could explain I really didn't drink much, he exclaimed, "I have been saving this wine for 12 years. I'm so happy I have the occasion to share it with you now!" Late in the meal, I looked up at Manu's face. He had tears running down it. He explained that he loved his family so much and he was so fortunate to be sitting there sharing his food with everyone. My eyes sprinkled, as well.

They knew I had had the gastric bypass, that I could only eat small portions. Yet we had the love of one another and our time together to celebrate.

There is a story by the author, Leo Buscaglia that I especially love. He told of his youth in Italy. On one occasion, his father came home early and told his wife and children that he had just lost his job. As he recounted his story and despaired of what would befall the family, Leo's mother quietly set the table with their good linens and dishes and then began to cook an elaborate meal. She made enough food for a feast.

Finally, Leo's father stopped his monologue and regarded his wife. "What are you doing, woman?" he asked. "I am telling you we are poor. We won't have money. Why are you cooking all this food?" "Because," said his wife, "the time for joy is now!"

And that, of course, is the point. The time for joy is always right now. Given the proverbial "second chance at life," I feel we owe ourselves a debt. We have abused our bodies with food. We have dampened our spirits with isolation. Now it is time for a life of meaning and celebration. Why shouldn't we enjoy, in any way we can, each and every moment? Realistically regard the negative of a situation, yes, but then address the positive in it, see the life lessons and move on to solution.

I read in an article that prisoners need to stand and wait for a guard to open a door. It is a barrier. Often, after their releases from prison, those who have been incarcerated a long time have become so accustomed to seeing themselves jailed they still hesitate before a door.

The closed doors from obesity don't have to remain shut to us. We can regain our health and become more emotionally expansive in the world. Venture out and explore it!

A favorite day for me is when I prepare a picnic lunch, put my camera in the car, choose a direction and just go. No expectations of what the day should hold or where I will end up.

I have discovered so many fascinating places just by driving into a town and asking a local person, "What is interesting about your town?" People, I find, are often anxious to become their town's ambassador. I have found treasures in little out of the way places I would have otherwise passed by.

And, as each door opens, the way is cleared to be receptive to what comes next. My friend, Sarah, has the same philosophy. She bought a sweatshirt and had the word "NEXT!" emblazoned on the front. If she were disappointed in a new love, she would pass her hand across her chest and yell, "Next!"

No moss grew on that lady!

Your Sweet Spirit

There is a concept that my friend, Tessie, in her wisdom, taught me. When we enter a new situation, we bring with us our sweet spirit. In so doing, we enhance the workplace or the relationship or the gathering. When we leave, we take that sweet spirit with us, as well, and that situation is now devoid of it.

Can you see your own sweet spirit that you bring to all you do? Can you see yourself as the gift? Interesting to think of yourself that way, isn't it? That just by your presence you are contributing so much. Think of that when you enter a new situation. As you ring the doorbell, the gift you are giving is your sweet spirit!

At Last Free

When I lost weight, I decided to do all the things in life that I thought my obesity had precluded me from doing.

For instance, my friend, Carl, enjoyed walking and he invited me along on his walks. We would walk and talk for hours and he would explain how the stock market worked.

Since he knew I had just lost a great deal of weight, he was comfortable asking me why I chose to join him on such longs walks of 15 miles a day. "Because I can," I told him.

And when I was in Florida, I signed up to swim with the manatees. I donned a wetsuit, walked onto a boat, lowered myself underwater and swam with these gentle and docile, gorgeous creatures. If it had been possible to cry under water from sheer joy, I would have.

One year, having read Shirley MacLaine's books on her experiences in Macchu Picchu, Peru's fortress city, I decided I would like to travel there to celebrate my weight loss and to find the spiritual connection described in her books. A week later, I entered a health food store and a flyer on the wall caught my eye. There was a tour group leaving on a trip to Peru. I smiled. I decided to take the flyer as a sign from Above that I was to go to South America. Two weeks later, I was standing 15,000 feet above sea level in the Andes.

Our group traveled with tour guides and a local shaman, Willaru, which means messenger. When my birthday fell, the shaman asked me how I would like to celebrate it. I told him I would like an evening of his time as my gift. We sat in the lodge, in front of a fire, while he told me about his life, his teachings and his philosophies. What an extraordinary exchange we had!

On the morning of the summer solstice, our group joined Willaru on the top of Macchu Pichu in the dark. He brought with him many ceremonial items, one of which was a huge, round crystal bowl. As the dawn peeked over the Andes, he repeatedly struck the bowl with a wooden mallet. The sound reverberated from one mountain to another. As we looked into the rising sun we were enveloped in sounds that penetrated our bodies. Tears filled our eyes. We thanked the Apus, the mountain gods, for allowing our presence and we danced. No food that I have ever eaten has tasted as good as my feelings from that memory.

Another year, my daughter and I planned a trip to Ireland. I was urged to get in touch with a physics professor at the University of Florida before my trip. He had been stationed in Ireland during World War II, had married an Irish woman and he settled there for many years afterward. I called him at home, explaining my desire to create a trip that had a strong spiritual base, while my daughter, Jennifer, an English Literature major, wanted to pursue a path leading her to the great writers and poets of Ireland. The professor invited me to his home and autographed my copy of the book he had written about the spiritual side of Ireland. On the map I brought, he drew the areas we should visit to get what each of us wanted from our adventure. As a consequence of his generous advice, we found what we needed in Ireland. We drove around all of the country, which included singing heartily in a pub in Doolin, the home of Irish folk music.

I have more stories of driving around England and of touring Israel, the United States, Peru and France. The point is, climbing up Masada or the Eiffel Tower would have been painful, maybe impossible, at 325 pounds. But a healthy, agile body allows me to pursue my dreams. Your good health will allow you your heart's desires, too.

Promises Fulfilled

When you were obese did you make promises to yourself? Did they go something like:

"When I lose weight I am going to............?"

"As soon as I'm thin I will..........?"

"I wish I could wake up thin so I can.................?"

Did you put life on hold until the Weight Loss Fairy would grant you a miracle? I certainly did.

There is an Irish song called The Parting Song (*Journey's End*). It's about a man who chooses a life of wandering, never committing to anyone, never fulfilling his promises to himself. The last verse goes:

"And when I'm done with wandering,

I will sit beside the road and weep.

For all the songs I did not sing

And for promises I did not keep [20]

I pray you sing all of your songs.

ACTION LIST

➢ Make a list of all the activities your weight has denied you doing.

➢ Love the life you have and make your dreams come true.

18

Sexual Feelings After
Weight Loss

"The most precious possession that ever comes to a man in this world is a woman's heart."

– Josiah G. Holland

"To love and be loved is to feel the sun from both sides."

– David Viscott

"All you need is love."

– John Lennon

Jerry was a member of a weight loss support group that I led. He spoke about being a chubby teenager and how he had put on a considerable amount of weight by the time he was 16. He indicated he had dated only once then and that he didn't feel comfortable asking girls out after that as he became more and more embarrassed about his size. He didn't attend his high school prom. He didn't date through college, or during his twenties or thirties either. He was shy and uncomfortable around women and conversation was difficult. By the time he underwent gastric bypass surgery at age 40, he had not developed much socially. When he substituted food for people, he lost the emotional development that social interaction would have taught him.

There was a time in childhood, for instance, when our friends were learning to ride a bike. If we learned along with them, then we took the falls as a natural course. Later, even if we hadn't ridden for years, we still retained the skills. However, if we never learned to ride as kids, it would be more frightening and embarrassing to learn to bike ride as an adult.

Jerry felt awkward and inept. He knew he was missing out on many wonderful experiences in life. And, he was terribly, miserably alone. He got up the courage one night to ask the group about how to begin meeting people. He had tears in his eyes and we understood his pain and fear. It was the opening for support from the group resulting in a lively discussion. All of us have had some or all of his experiences. He shared his feelings. We listened. We shared ours. He realized he wasn't alone in this situation.

He soon became the leader of the After-Support-Group, Let's-Go-Out-For-Decaf-Coffee-Club. The support group became a place for the learning of new social skills and was, thus, a valuable asset.

Of superior value in a good support group is social interaction. When we have a common reason to be in the room, it is easier to strike up a conversation. Ask a question that may require another person to elaborate. Listen well. People like to talk about themselves, their achievements, where they are on their weight loss path. I find conversation quickly comfortable at support group. We all "know" each other's lives from the standpoint of having suffered with the same disease. I find people reveal intimate parts of their lives in the support group environment that they wouldn't dream of sharing in some other milieu. Dating and marriages have resulted from meeting people in support group. Support group allows you to turn to the group at the end of the evening and to invite everyone out for further socializing and thus allows a safe group environment in which to practice new social skills.

Sexual Advances

As the weight comes off, the body is unveiled. We notice new contours and signals from others that our bodies are becoming more sexually appealing. This revelation can incite feelings ranging from eager anticipation to abject terror.

"For some of us, body weight acts as a shield giving us a feeling of protection from sexual abuse or from intimacy. Extra weight seems to be a way to take the body out of the market. We aren't burdened with having to be measured against others or with having to compete for attention from the opposite sex. We feel safe from rejection, as if we have chosen to reject others first."[3]

Much of our assumption that the weight will render us too unattractive to be loved by others is just a myth. If you look around you will see many overweight people are very attractive and they have active social lives. When walking down the street, I have seen slender men holding hands with "heavy" women and I have seen, slender women with obese men. Do we think all people dating and making love and marrying are beanpoles? It is not the weight that renders us unattractive. We are unavailable because we have learned to give signals to others that we are closed to their intimacy both emotionally and physically.

Part of learning to live in a normal weighted body, also, is realizing you have the power to choose or reject sexual advances by your words. "No," as the saying goes, "is a complete sentence." No is a good word to learn, for you do not have to tolerate someone else's advances upon your body. You no longer have to abuse yourself with food to feel safe, nor do you have to say yes to an invitation, to feel loved and accepted, as many obese women have done.

Some of us want to explore relationship, but the fear keeps sabotaging our efforts. It will ease your way if you find activities you enjoy doing and meet other people enjoying them, too.

Beware The Sexual Predator

At the other end of the spectrum is the person who has felt so left out of social interaction, so powerless, that he feels he needs the "whole candy store," so to speak, of sexual opportunities.

Suppose the man was very heavy in college and women wouldn't date him. Now he may want to "catch up" on all those years of deprivation of female attention. Since 80% of gastric bypass patients are women, a typical weight loss support group, by its very nature, is filled with women who may have not developed good emotional boundaries and skills for interacting with others. It can be an easy place for the man to "hit on all the ladies," but consider this if you are a man: is it fair to prey sexually on someone who hasn't learned the skills to defend herself? Is that who you want to be?

At one group I led, there was a man who had previously weighed 600 pounds and who now weighed in the 200's. Even though he was married and his wife frequently came to the group to support him, he approached several women for sexual liaisons, including me. I strongly urged him to seek professional counseling before he destroyed a relationship with his loving wife, who had stuck with him through thick and thin – literally.

Our challenge is to learn the meaning of the nonverbal signals of others. Is this person just being friendly or is there a stronger motive behind the action? Without experience it is hard to measure a person's intent. Practice, along with feedback, help us grow.

Intimacy

Now is the time to get to know yourself better.

- How would you describe yourself at your current age?

- What do you want from relationships now?

- What is realistic sexual function for your age?

- Is it better to avoid an intimate relationship for the first year of weight loss while you are working on your emotional issues?

- Do you want to explore the possibility of real intimacy for the first time in your life?

- Is it frightening to pull someone close?

I ask these questions about intimacy because it can be a tricky topic. Most of us haven't had a lot of experience with being truly intimate with others. Remember, we have practiced substitution for intimacy and avoidance of relationship for years. Sometimes we pull people close to us on the one hand and, on the other hand, push them away with behavior that signals we don't want them to come close. The landmines we plant will confuse, injure and dissuade the recipient from truly opening her heart. If you can't figure out why the person you claim to love often pulls away from you, ask yourself if you are planting these landmines to destroy intimacy.

The new you is emerging. Mold and create the person you want to be and teach other people who you are.

Changes in sexual patterns after surgery are common. People report an increase in frequency, quality and in their enjoyment of sex. As body image improves there is often an improvement in sexual functioning, as well.

Interesting to note, however, some people report for months after surgery that their interest in sex is diminished and it is not at all unusual.

ACTION LIST

➢ Attend a weight loss support group.

➢ On your list of pleasurable alternatives to food, add a new activity to meet people whose interests match your own.

➢ Get advice in choosing new clothes from someone whose taste you trust. Get a massage. Get a facial. Exercise to strengthen your body. Do something to challenge your mind. Stay apprised of current events. Form opinion. Connect with the world in a way that will salve your spirit. The increased self-esteem will be evident to yourself and to others.

➢ Accept invitations from friends. You never know where you will meet someone.

➢ Be the one to strike up a conversation. What's the worst that can happen?

➢ If all of this is too frightening for you, see a therapist who will support you in your efforts to gain your social footing in the world.

19

Gratitude:
Giving Something Back

"Gratitude is not only the greatest of virtues, but the parent of all others."

– Cicero (106BC-43BC) Pro Plancio, 54BC

To Tell Or Not To Tell

I have been asked many times in weight loss support groups whether I think the participant should tell people outside of the group about her surgery. I would never recommend telling if, to do so, places you in a truly vulnerable position. After all, we are trying to raise self-esteem, not to defeat ourselves. Each of us decides this issue for herself.

But if you are comfortable and you can offer relief to the suffering of another human being, I say reveal yourself because almost everyone these days has an obese loved one or friend. It is part of learning to be open about one's life. In 12-step Programs, they say, "You are only as sick as your secrets."

I know I have stored food like a squirrel facing winter, eaten at secret places and hidden my "identity" from the world. The ironic discovery for me was in realizing that the more open and disclosing I was, the safer I felt. No one can "find out" about me what I have already revealed myself. I am human. I have made mistakes. I am learning.

Recovery requires me to create a confluence of thought on the inside, with my actions on the outside. I create a conflict in living if this confluence does not take place. Honesty is crucial to my weight loss program.

"You cannot divide your brain. You must choose integrity in all areas of your life. I often speak on the issue of integrity because I've learned that dishonesty begins with food and then spreads throughout your character.

"Lie about your surgery, be dishonest about your surgery, hide your surgery, all of these things are detrimental to your weight loss maintenance. Your character suffers from each deception. Every lie eats away at your integrity and ultimately your Being. The body is an outward manifestation of the mind. Lies and deceit will reveal themselves in places that feed our shame and embarrassment—most of us call that place: 'Our waist'. Honesty within is worn without.

Instead of falling tongue-tied, imagine if the next time someone asked you what you did to lose weight, you could make eye contact, smile and, using one or two sentences, convey just the right words to answer with integrity and candor:

'I had weight loss surgery. It was the best decision I ever made to change my body and my mind. I am happy and healthy for the first time in decades.'"[19]

We are a world connected and our actions affect others with far-reaching results. You will feel "cleaner" in life if you deal honestly with others about your "new you".

Gratitude

The ebb and flow of life requires us to take in and to give back. How could we help but be eternally grateful for a surgery that has helped us to achieve such cosmetic improvement and good health? I practice gratitude for my fortune everyday, saying thank you for my new life of health in some manner. There is just something about gratitude that gives me a generous-hearted outlook on life.

Gratitude can be expressed in a thousand ways. Extend your arms out to the world. Smile at people you meet in your day. Encourage others. Listen well. Say thank you for people's effort in your behalf and for their time. Be a friend.

At a recent bariatric convention, I walked up to my surgeon whom I haven't seen since I had surgery almost five years ago. I introduced myself and told him how he had impacted my life. "Thank you", I said, "for giving me back my life and for giving me the chance to fulfill my purpose." Ours eyes were watery.

In the hospital where I worked, I wrote a sensitivity program on behalf of the patients who would utilize the facility. I went around to every department to speak with the employees about the disease of obesity and about how we could make our incoming patients feel more welcome and accepted. It was my way to express my gratitude for a second chance at life and renewed health.

ACTION LIST

➢ Decide how you can express your gratitude for getting a second chance at life.

---

[20]

Containing Joy

"When death comes and whispers to me,
'Thy days are ended,'
let me say to him, 'I have lived in love and not in mere time.'
He will ask, 'Will thy songs remain?'
I shall say, 'I know not, but this I know
That often when I sang I found my eternity."

Tagore (Fireflies)

People have expressed to me they feel they will regain the weight and lose the new joy they have attained and, so, they set out to sabotage their efforts before "life does them in." They are accustomed to seeing themselves fail and their new joy feels strange and oddly uncomfortable. If they have a minor setback, if life doesn't always go their way, they lapse into the anticipation of failure.

There is a concept in Chinese philosophy that teaches us to contain joy, that is, to put it in perspective. This does not mean that you must stifle joy in any way. It merely tells us that all of life is yin and yang, ebb and flow, joy and sorrow and that the joy we are now feeling will, as in all things in our lives, pass and be replaced temporarily with whatever comes next.

We do not live in a state of continuous joy. Our lives are not ecstatic experiences, strung one after the other. Golden moments, yes, hopefully we will have many, but not a constant state of joy. We learn from all of our experiences and it is in seeing the shadow of life that we appreciate the sunshine to its fullest.

Struggle is necessary for growth. "Friction is a fundamental property of nature and nothing grows without it– not mountains, not pearls, not people. It is precisely the quality of fragility, the capacity for being 'shaken up', that is paradoxically the key to growth. Any structure that is insulated from disturbance is also protected from change.

We must, therefore, be willing to be shaken up, to submit ourselves to the dark blossomings of chaos, in order to reap the blessings of growth."[21]

Have you ever read about celebrities who, seemingly, have it all? They have attained fame, beauty and fortune, far beyond what most of us imagine for ourselves. Nonetheless, they find a way to subvert it, to bring it down. They commit crimes that ruin their reputations. They create relationships that result in divorce after divorce. They spend money recklessly. They commit suicide. Why waste the gift of life?

Joy, as sorrow, is a golden strand that weaves in and out of the tapestry of our lives, but it is not our total fabric. We would still be ourselves without fame. We would still be ourselves without wealth. Our beauty fades. We have only our character, our core, and our essence as solid, steadfast, defined. It is in taking these joyful experiences in stride, knowing they will change course again, that we gain power.

On the other hand, some people fear that joy is something too transitory and fleeting, not deserved and too good to believe. We may feel overwhelmed by it.

Recidivism is not inevitable. I recognize that it has been our pattern. Yet there are people who have had gastric bypass surgery over 20 years ago and they are normal weight and healthy. You have a new tool. Stay calm in the joy of a new body, believe in yourself, protect your program from the sabotage of others, stay the course. In time you will have confidence that success is gained by merely working calmly in the day to day and that you are doing just that.

Life for you will be about keeping your program sacred, dealing with past memories and also in living in the today of your life. Surround yourself with people who help you to believe in yourself. This is your work. Your burden of excess weight is gone and you have the opportunity to express yourself in a new way. You have the opportunity to create new life.

...and you have been taught to fly.

Final Note

I sincerely hope this book was of value to you.

Having begun my second book on obesity, I invite you to e-mail me your story. I want to hear about your life, how obesity has impacted it, and what your journey has been. Perhaps you have had humorous moments along the way. Maybe your struggle has been tough, but it will show others how you persevered and overcame problems. If I include your story in my book, I will do so with great care maintaining your anonymity and privacy, of course. Likewise, your e-mail address will never, ever be given out, rented or sold to anyone else.

Let me know about your tears, triumphs and joy! E-mail me your thoughts to peckpublishing@yahoo.com.

My second book will deal with more of an in depth understanding of the aftermath of surgery, how to get the most from the pouch, the disease of morbid obesity itself and more long term strategies.

My best,

Paula

Appendices

Appendix A

IBSR Medical Advisory Committee, November 2001.
Complications Within 30 Days Of Surgical Treatment For
Obesity

No complication	10,241	93.16
Minor:*		
other: drug skin problems, balloon dilatation, hemorrhoidectomy, gastroenteritis, undefined	165	1.50
atelectasis (46), hyperventilation (1), respiratory undefined (104)	151	1.37
wound site seroma (80), wound infection (48)	128	1.17
splenic injury	27	0.25
pleural effusion (11), pleuritis (2), pneumonitis (9),	22	0.20
dehydration	8	0.07
renal, urinary tract infection (4)	7	0.06
stoma too large (5), stoma too small (1)	6	0.05
ulcers: duodenal, gastric, stomal (jejunum or anastomoses)	5	0.05
hepatic, liver hematoma (1)	4	0.04
esophageal reflux, esophagitis (2)	3	0.03
hernia: incisional (1), ventral (1)	2	0.02
dumping syndrome (1), vitamin insufficiency (1)	2	0.02
Major: *		
GI Leak (*5 deaths*)	33	0.30
stoma obstruction (lumenal - 18); stoma stenosis (15)	33	0.30
GI hemorrhage or GI bleeding; 7 due to ulcers,	26	0.24

undefined (19)		
cardiac (*4 deaths*)	19	0.17
pulmonary embolism (*11 deaths*)	19	0.17
respiratory arrest or failure (*4 deaths*)	16	0.15
wound dehiscence	13	0.12
small bowel obstruction: Roux-en-y (4), common channel (2), enterostomy (1) undefined (6)	13	0.12
subphrenic / subhepatic abscess; abdominal abscess (1)	11	0.10
gastric dilatation (*1 death*)	11	0.10
deep venous thrombosis (6), thrombophlebitis (2)	8	0.07
stapleline breakdown: linear gastric (3), window (1), enterostomy (3 - *2 deaths*)	7	0.06
pancreatitis (3); acute cholecystitis (2)	5	0.05
neurologic (*1 death*)	4	0.04
gastric fistula	3	0.03
peritonitis (*2 deaths*)	2	0.02
Total Patients	10,993	100.00

Appendix B

Body Mass index (BMI) Chart

<18.5 (Underweight) 18.5-24.9 (Normal) 25-29.9 (Overweight) 30-34.9 (Obese I) 35-39.9 (Obese II) >40 (Mortbidly Obese)

Weight (in pounds)

HEIGHT (ft/in)	120	130	140	150	160	170	180	190	200	210	220	230	240	250	260	270	280	290	300	310	320
4'10"	25	27	29	31	34	36	38	40	42	44	46	48	50	52	54	57	59	61	63	65	67
4'11"	24	26	28	30	32	34	36	38	40	43	45	47	49	51	53	55	57	59	61	63	65
5'0"	23	25	27	29	31	33	35	37	39	41	43	45	47	49	51	53	55	57	59	61	63
5'1"	23	25	27	28	30	32	34	36	38	40	42	44	45	47	49	51	53	55	57	59	61
5'2"	22	24	26	27	29	31	33	35	37	38	40	42	44	46	48	49	51	53	55	57	59
5'3"	21	23	25	27	28	30	32	34	36	37	39	41	43	44	46	48	50	51	53	55	57
5'4"	21	22	24	26	28	29	31	33	34	36	38	40	41	43	45	46	48	50	52	53	55
5'5"	20	22	23	25	27	28	30	32	33	35	37	38	40	42	43	45	47	48	50	52	53
5'6"	19	21	23	24	26	27	29	31	32	34	36	37	39	40	42	44	45	47	49	50	52
5'7"	19	20	22	24	25	27	28	30	31	33	35	36	38	39	41	42	44	46	47	49	50
5'8"	18	20	21	23	24	26	27	29	30	32	34	35	37	38	40	41	43	44	46	47	49
5'9"	18	19	21	22	24	25	27	28	30	31	33	34	36	37	38	40	41	43	44	46	47
5'10"	17	19	20	22	23	24	26	27	29	30	32	33	35	36	37	39	40	42	43	45	46

Weight (in pounds)

	120	130	140	150	160	170	180	190	200	210	220	230	240	250	260	270	280	290	300	310	320
5'11"	17	18	20	21	22	24	25	27	28	29	31	32	34	35	36	38	39	41	42	43	45
6'0"	16	18	19	20	22	23	24	26	27	29	30	31	33	34	35	37	38	39	41	42	43
6'1"	16	17	19	20	21	22	24	25	26	28	29	30	32	33	34	36	37	38	40	41	42
6'2"	15	17	18	19	21	22	23	24	26	27	28	30	31	32	33	35	36	37	39	40	41

APPENDIX C

WEIGHT LOSS PROGRESS CHART

MONTH_____ DAY_____ YEAR_____

WEIGHT

EXERCISE
WATER
VITAMINS

Appendix D

Plastic Surgery

It is with great pleasure I recommend Dr. Alexander Sinclair, Plastic Surgeon. Dr. Sinclair loves to perform surgery to help formerly obese patients. His address is 9675 Brighton Way, #410, Beverly Hills, CA 90210. Don't let the Beverly Hills address scare you. Dr. Sinclair offers fair fees combined with meticulous surgical work. He is calm, humble, and respectful. He understands the bariatric patient and deals deftly with contouring the once-obese body. I flew across the country so he would be my doctor. I'm glad I did.

His telephone number is (310) 274-4103. His Web site is www.alexandersinclairmd.com.

References

[1] American Society for Bariatric Surgery. *Surgery For Morbid Obesity: What Patients Should Know.*

[2] First Magazine

[3] Katherine, Anne. *Anatomy of a Food Addiction, The Brain Chemistry of Overeating.* Gurze Books,

[4] Gaye Andrews, Ph.D. *Living a Lighter Lifestyle.*

[5] National Institutes of Health. News Release, June, 1988.

[6] National Institute of Health. Statistical study.

[7] The American Society for Bariatric Surgery cites the Framingham study in their rationale for having the gastric bypass surgery:

[8] Drs. Clark and Whitgrove.. *Laparoscopic Operations.* Center for Surgical Weight Control. San Diego, CA

[9] Deitel, Mervyn M.D. Surgery For the Morbidly Obese Patient. Lea and Febiger, 1989

[10] National Institutes of Health

[11] Wald, Erica. *Psychological Aspects of Gastric Bypass Surgery.*

[12] Dr. Musante, Durham, North Carolina.

[13] American Society of Bariatric Surgeons. *Surgery for Morbid Obesity.*

[14] This analogy suggested by Leslie Jester, RN, San Diego, CA.

[15] Brownell, Kelly D. Ph.D. *Learn Program of Weight Management 2000.* Yale University

[16] Beyond Change

[17] Viscott, David M.D. Emotionally Free: Letting Go of the Past to Live in the Moment. Contemporary Books, 1992.

[18] Andrews, Gaye Ph.D. *Living a Lighter Lifestyle, A Guide to Successful Weight Loss and Maintenance Following Gastroplasty or Gastric Bypass.* Wheat Field Publications, 1994.

[19] Holtzclaw, Teri Kai Ph.D. This is Not Brain Surgery,

[20] Goodenough, J.B. "Journey's End." Bucks Music

[21] Levoy, Gregg. *Callings.* Three Rivers Press. New York, 1997

Bibliography

Viscott, David M.D. Emotionally Free: Letting Go of the Past to Live in the Moment. Contemporary Books, 1992.

Andrews, Gaye Ph.D. *Living a Lighter Lifestyle, A Guide to SuccessfulWeight Loss and Maintenance Following Gastroplasty or Gastric Bypass.* Wheat Field Publications, 1994.

Vista Medical Technologies, Alvarado Center for Surgical Weight Control. *The Laparoscopic Bariatric Surgery Program.* 2001

Katherine M. Flegal; Margaret D. Carroll; Cynthia L. Ogden; Clifford L. Johnson. "Prevalence and Trends in Obesity Among US Adults, 1999-2000." *JAMA.* 2002;288:1723-1727.

Beyond Change. JKS Associates. Bloomfield Hills, MI.

Holtzclaw, Teri Kai, Ph. D. *This is NOT Brain Surgery! A Mental Health Companion for the Gastric Bypass Patient.* MorrisPublishing, 1997.

Katherine, Anne. *Anatomy of a Food Addiction, The Brain Chemistryof Overeating.* Gurze Books, 1991

Goodenough, J.B. "Journey's End." Bucks Music

Edmund J. Bourne. *The Anxiety and Phobia Workbook.* New Harbinger Publications, 1995.

Eades, Michael M.D. Eades, Mary Dan M.D. *The Protein Power Lifeplan.* Warner Books, 2000

Deitel, Mervyn M.D. *Surgery For the Morbidly Obese Patient.* Lea and Febiger, 1989

Brownell, Kelly D. Ph.D. *The Learn Program for Weight Management 2000.* American Health, 2000.

Internet Resources

American Diabetes Association
www.diabetes.org

American Heart Association
www.americanheart.org

American Medical Association (AMA)
www.ama-assn.org

American Obesity Association
www.obesity.org

American Society for Bariatric Surgery (ASBS)
www.asbs.org

American Society of Bariatric Physicians
www.asbp.org

Association for Morbid Obesity Support
www.obesityhelp.com Obesityhelp.com

Beyond Change
www.beyondchange-obesity.com

Eating Disorders Awareness and Prevention, Inc. (EDAP)
www.edap.org

International Bariatric Surgery Registry
www.surgery.uiowa.edu/nbsr/ibsrbroc.html

M.O.R.E. Foundation (Morbid Obesity Research Efforts)
www.morefoundation.org

National Heart, Lung, and Blood Institute
www.nhlbi.nih.gov

North American Association for the Study of Obesity
www.naaso.org

Obesity-Online
www.obesity-online.com

Weight-control Information Network
www.niddk.nih.gov/health/nutrit/win.htm

INDEX

A

alcohol, 133

anesthesiologist, 28

B

behavioral changes, 70

bingeing, 146, 186

BMI, 25

C

carbohydrates, 21, 62

celebrating, 193

co-morbidities, 17, 26, 29

constipation, 73

D

Dear Me Letter, 33, 37

depression, 19, 35, 50, 72, 146, 147, 153

diabetes, 15, 16, 25, 75, 128

diet head, 82

dieting, 19, 21

digestive system, 44

dispelling old beliefs, 141, 148, 151

Dumping Syndrome, 45, 57, 63

E

education, 35

ethnic foods, 132

exercise, 84, 96, 105, 109, 111, 112

F

fat prejudice, 159

final pigout, 38

food buffets, 136

food triggers, 129

fun, 51, 72, 76, 84, 100, 105, 110, 139, 183, 185, 196

G

gastric bypass, 8, 44

GERD, 70

golden period, 68

guided imagery, 114

H

hair loss, 87

holidays, 139

honeymoon period, 55

hunger, 79

hypertension, 25

I

image perception, 173

initial consultation, 27

insurance, 25

J

journaling, 51, 63, 64, 74, 77, 98, 99, 182

joy, 215

L

laparoscopic surgery, 20, 38, 50

laparotomy, 45

lifestyle changes, 20, 83, 90, 125, 133

M

massage, 110

morbid obesity, 15, 26

P

parties, 136

pregnancy, 29

primary foods, 131

protein foods, 87

psychologist, 7, 36, 105, 176

R

restaurants, 134

restructuring relationships, 167

Roux-en-Y, 8, 29, 43, 45

S

salad bars, 136

self-defeat, 91

sex, 201

six months and beyond, 79

sleep apnea, 46

snacking, 62, 73, 84, 87, 90

social skills, 151

spirometer, 51

sugar substances, 58

supermarket shopping, 126, 143

support, 35

support group, 36, 97

surgery

    day before, 46

    day of discharge, 50

    honeymoon period, 55

    six months and beyond, 81

    surgery day - postop, 48

    surgery day - preop, 47

    three to six months, 68

surgical athlete, 36

T

target heart rate, 120

The Wave, 134

traveling, 140

V

vitamins, 36, 85

vomiting, 57, 69

W

walking, 36, 50, 100, 105, 108, 109, 114

weighing yourself, 72

Weight Loss Surgery. *See* gastric bypass

For orders please go to:

Bariatric Advantage Vitamins at:

<u>www.bariatricadvantage.com</u>

Amazon at:

<u>www.amazon.com</u>